Handbook of Dermatologic Surgery

Handbook of Dermatologic Surgery

Elizabeth Hale, M.D.
New York University of School of Medicine
New York, NY, USA

Julie Karen, M.D.
New York University of School of Medicine
New York, NY, USA

Perry Robins, M.D.
New York University of School of Medicine
New York, NY, USA

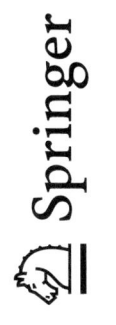

Springer

Elizabeth Hale
New York University School of Medicine
New York, NY, USA

Perry Robins
New York University School of Medicine
New York, NY, USA

Julie Karen
New York University School of Medicine
New York, NY, USA

ISBN 978-1-4614-8334-2 ISBN 978-1-4614-8335-9 (eBook)
DOI 10.1007/978-1-4614-8335-9
Springer New York Heidelberg Dordrecht London

Library of Congress Control Number: 2013951514

© Springer Science+Business Media New York 2014

This work is subject to copyright. All rights are reserved by the Publisher, whether the whole or part of the material is concerned, specifically the rights of translation, reprinting, reuse of illustrations, recitation, broadcasting, reproduction on microfilms or in any other physical way, and transmission or information storage and retrieval, electronic adaptation, computer software, or by similar or dissimilar methodology now known or hereafter developed. Exempted from this legal reservation are brief excerpts in connection with reviews or scholarly analysis or material supplied specifically for the purpose of being entered and executed on a computer system, for exclusive use by the purchaser of the work. Duplication of this publication or parts thereof is permitted only under the provisions of the Copyright Law of the Publisher's location, in its current version, and permission for use must always be obtained from Springer. Permissions for use may be obtained through RightsLink at the Copyright Clearance Center. Violations are liable to prosecution under the respective Copyright Law.

The use of general descriptive names, registered names, trademarks, service marks, etc. in this publication does not imply, even in the absence of a specific statement, that such names are exempt from the relevant protective laws and regulations and therefore free for general use.

While the advice and information in this book are believed to be true and accurate at the date of publication, neither the authors nor the editors nor the publisher can accept any legal responsibility for any errors or omissions that may be made. The publisher makes no warranty, express or implied, with respect to the material contained herein.

Springer is part of Springer Science+Business Media (www.springer.com)

Foreword

Dermatologic surgery has become a very important part of dermatology and includes a wide range of procedures from biopsies to advanced reconstructive, oncologic, and cosmetic surgeries. Additionally, dramatically expanding applications of lasers and light sources have increased the role of these devices in the field of dermatology. Patients will expect their dermatologist to perform many of these procedures. This handbook offers a practical, yet comprehensive, overview of common dermatologic procedures. Besides incorporating the basics of cutaneous oncology and dermatologic surgery, this book also superbly explores laser surgery and other subspecialties related to the field. The chapters in this book run the gamut from the everyday procedures carried out by the general dermatologist to the more advanced techniques carried out by the leaders of our field.

Handbook of dermatologic surgery is a comprehensive handbook that incorporates instructive concepts of the procedures involved in the modern practice of dermatologic surgery and procedural dermatology and is a resource that will be beneficial to not only those engaged in the field of dermatologic surgery but also residents and medical students seeking knowledge on performing these procedures. The book begins with the basics of dermatologic surgery such as suture techniques and progresses to more advanced procedures including reconstructions, lasers, and cosmetic dermatology.

Foreword

"Observing" and thereby familiarizing oneself with the key concepts presented in this book is only the first step towards acquiring expertise in dermatologic surgery. The next step, of course, is "doing." It is by observing and doing something over and over again that we become masters of the technique. May you find this a useful tool in your furtherance of dermatologic surgery education.

It has been a privilege to work on this book with Drs. Elizabeth Hale and Julie Karen, two sisters and dermatologists extraordinaire. As Professor Emeritus of Dermatology at NYU Langone Medical Center, and the first Mohs surgeon east of the Mississippi, the teaching of dermatologic surgery has always been my mission and true passion. I know Liz and Julie will follow my footsteps and continue to advance the future of dermatologic surgery.

New York, NY, USA   Perry Robins, M.D.

Acknowledgment

We would like to thank Jesse M. Lewin, M.D. for his input and assistance in putting this handbook together.

Table of Contents

Section A: Surgical Anatomy

Figure 1.1: Anterior view of the skull 1
Figure 1.2: Lateral view of the skull 2
Figure 1.3: Lateral view: muscles
of the head and neck 3
Figure 1.4: *Left*: branches of cranial nerve VII
(facial nerve), *Right*: sensory nerves
of the face 4
Table 1.1: Branches of cranial nerve V
(trigeminal nerve) 5
Figure 1.5: Branches of the facial nerve
(*circles* indicate areas at greatest
risk for injury)... 5
Figure 1.6: Vascular supply to the face 6
Figure 1.7: Anatomy of the nose................................. 7
Figure 1.8: Subunits of the face................................... 8
Figure 1.9: Anatomy of the external ear 9
Figure 1.10: Anatomy of the eye................................ 10
Figure 1.11: Anatomy of the nail unit........................ 11
Figure 1.12: Skin tension lines (*face*): for planning
optimal incisions to minimize scarring...... 12
Figure 1.13: Skin tension lines (anterior) 13
Figure 1.14: Skin tension lines (posterior) 14
Figure 1.15: Great saphenous vein (GSV)
and its tributaries...................................... 15
Figure 1.16: Small saphenous vein (SSV)
and its tributaries...................................... 16

ix

Table of Contents

Section B: Excisional and Non-excisional Surgery

- Preoperative History 17
- Figure 2.1: Guidelines for prophylactic and empiric antibiotics. 20
- Table 2.1: Commonly used prophylactic antibiotic agents for cutaneous surgery. 21
- Table 2.2: Antiseptic scrubs. 22
- Table 2.3: Local anesthetics. 23
- Anesthetics: Key Facts 25
- Table 2.4: Tumescent anesthesia solution. 27
- Table 2.5: Electrosurgery 28
- Cryosurgery. 30
- Table 2.6: Recommended surgical margins 32
- Table 2.7: Melanoma staging. 34
- Main Indications for Mohs Micrographic Surgery 38
- Mohs Micrographic Surgery Procedure 39
- Figure 2.2: Mohs micrographic surgery 40
- Elliptical Fusiform Excision 41
- Figure 2.3: Elliptical fusiform excision 41
- Placement of Incisions and Excisions on the Face 42
- Figure 2.4: Placement of incisions and excisions on the face. 42
- Simple Interrupted Stitch 43
- Figure 2.5: Simple interrupted stitch 43
- Buried Vertical Mattress Stitch. 44

Table of Contents

Figure 2.6: Buried vertical mattress stitch for deep dermal tissue approximation and eversion 44
Cutaneous Vertical Mattress Stitch 45
Figure 2.7: Vertical mattress stitch 45
Horizontal Mattress Stitch 46
Figure 2.8: (a, b) Horizontal mattress stitch 46
Running Subcuticular Stitch 47
Figure 2.9: Running subcuticular/intradermal stitch 47
Pulley Stitch 48
Figure 2.10: Pulley stitch (epidermal): for closure of wounds under tension 48
Three Point Suture (aka Tip stitch) 49
Figure 2.11: Three-point stitch (AKA tip stitch) 49
"Dog Ear" Repair 50
Figure 2.12: Repair of dog ears 50
"Leashing" of Dog Ears 51
Figure 2.13: "Leashing" the dog ear 52
Table 2.8: Absorbable sutures 53
Table 2.9: Nonabsorbable sutures 55
Table 2.10: Topical antimicrobial agents 56
Table 2.11: Wound dressing 58
Table 2.12: Surgical complications 59
Table 2.13: Suture removal timetable 63
Commonly Used Surgical Instruments in Dermatologic Surgery 64
Figure 2.14: Scalpel handles 64
Figure 2.15: Scalpel blades 65
Figure 2.16: Curettes 66
Figure 2.17: Needle holders 67
Figure 2.18: Adson Forceps 68
Figure 2.19: Bishop Harmon forceps 69

xi

Table of Contents

Figure 2.20: Jacobson hemostat forceps 70
Figure 2.21: Scissors: general operating scissors for suture cutting 71
Figure 2.22: Scissors: the curved Mayo scissor (*left*), and the straight Metzenbaum scissor with blunted tips (*right*) 72
Figure 2.23: Castroviejo needle driver 73
Figure 2.24: Chalazion clamp 74
Figure 2.25: Skin hook 75
Figure 2.26: English nail splitter 76
Figure 2.27: Nail elevator 77

Section C: Advanced Repairs

Flap Overview 79
Single Advancement Flap 80
Figure 3.1: Single advancement flap 80
Bilateral Advancement Flap (H-Plasty) 81
Figure 3.2: Bilateral advancement flap 81
Z-Plasty 82
Figure 3.3: Z-plasty 82
M-Plasty 83
Figure 3.4: M-plasty 83
Figure 3.5: M-plasty 84
S-Plasty 85
Figure 3.6: S-plasty 85
Rotation Flap 86
Figure 3.7: Rotation flap 86
Double Advancement Rotation Flap (O-Z Plasty) 87
Figure 3.8: Double advancement rotation flap or O-Z plasty 87
Rhomboid Flap 88
Figure 3.9: Standard rhomboid transposition flap, modified rhomboid flap 88

xii

Table of Contents

Bilobed Transposition Flap 89
Figure 3.10: (a): Traditional bilobed transposition flap, (b): Zitelli modified bilobed transposition flap 89
Skin Grafts Overview 90
Stages of Graft Survival 90
Table 3.1: Skin graft types 91

Section D: Cosmetic Dermatology: Fillers, Neurotoxins, and Chemical Peels

Table 4.1: Botulinum toxin dilutions 93
Table 4.2: Injectable fillers 94
Table 4.3: Chemical peels 98

Section E: Lasers and Other Technology

Laser Overview: Light Amplification by Stimulated Emission of Radiation 99
Table 5.1: Lasers used in dermatology 100
Table 5.2: Fractionated laser devices 104
Table 5.3: Home use and low-energy devices 106
Table 5.4: Tattoo removal by laser 108
Table 5.5: Photo-induced eye injury 110
Novel Devices: Skin Tightening and Body Sculpting 111

Section F: Leg Veins

Leg Vein Treatment Overview 113
Leg Vein Treatment Algorithm 115
Table 6.1: Laser for leg veins 116
Table 6.2: Sclerotherapy agents 117

Index 121

xiii

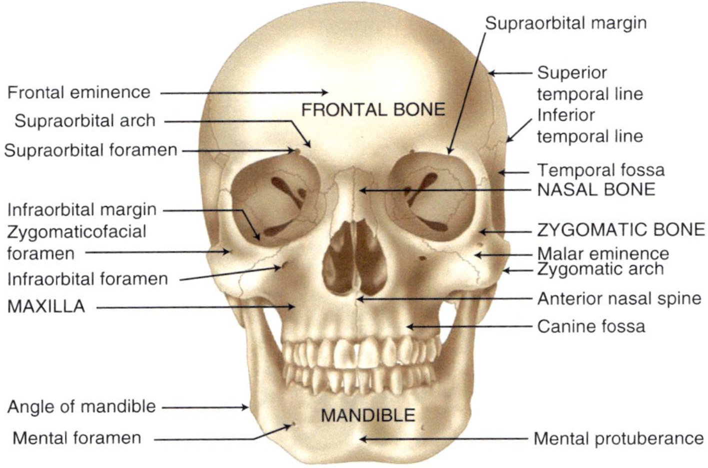

Section A Surgical Anatomy

Figure 1.1 Anterior view of the skull

E. Hale et al., *Handbook of Dermatologic Surgery*,
10.1007/978-1-4614-8335-9_1, © Springer Science+Business Media New York 2014

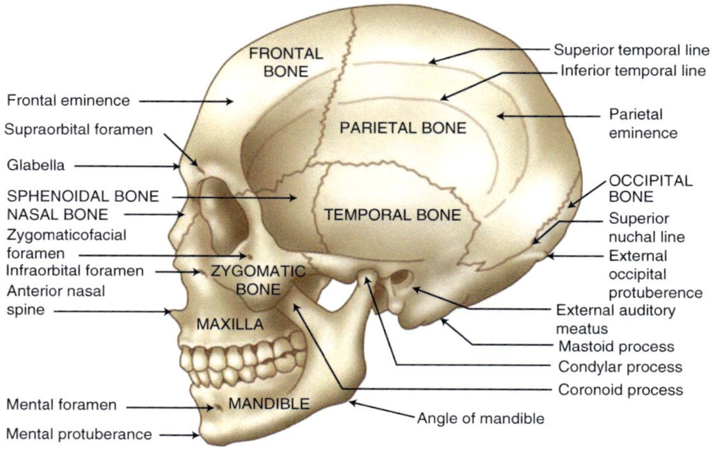

Section A   **Surgical Anatomy**

Figure 1.2 Lateral view of the skull

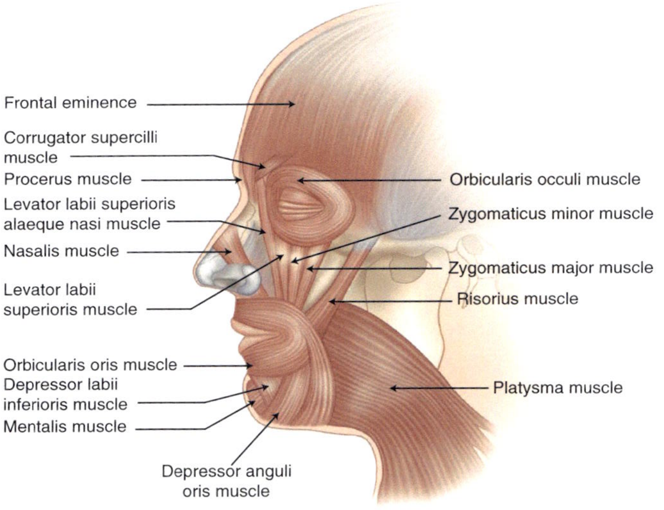

Section A Surgical Anatomy

Figure 1.3 Lateral view: muscles of the head and neck

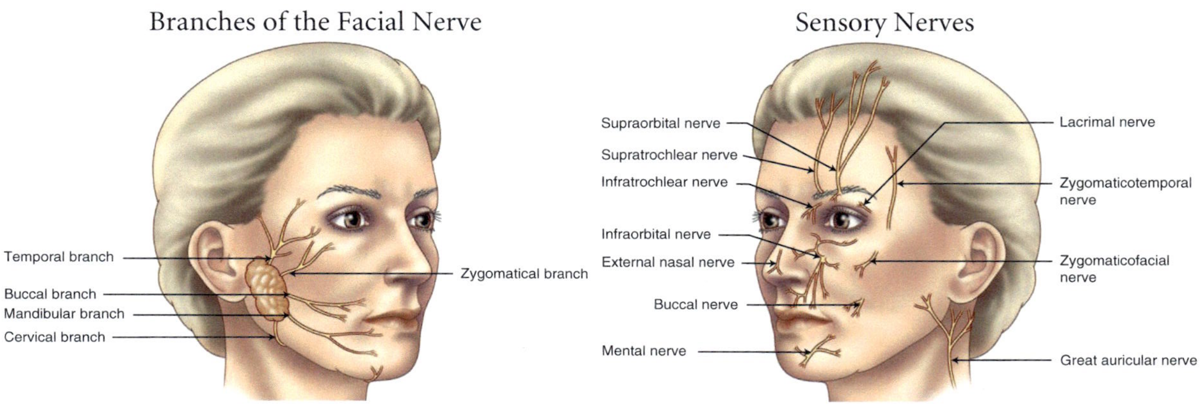

Section A Surgical Anatomy

Branches of the Facial Nerve

- Temporal branch
- Buccal branch
- Mandibular branch
- Cervical branch
- Zygomatical branch

Sensory Nerves

- Lacrimal nerve
- Zygomaticotemporal nerve
- Zygomaticofacial nerve
- Great auricular nerve
- Supraorbital nerve
- Supratrochlear nerve
- Infratrochlear nerve
- Infraorbital nerve
- External nasal nerve
- Buccal nerve
- Mental nerve

Figure 1.4 *Left*: branches of cranial nerve VII (facial nerve), *Right*: sensory nerves of the face

Section A Surgical Anatomy

V₁ ophthalmic
- Supraorbital nerve
- Supratrochlear nerve
- Infratrochlear nerve
- External nasal nerve
- Lacrimal nerve

V₂ maxillary
- Infraorbital nerve
- Zygomaticofacial nerve
- Zygomaticotemporal nerve

V₃ mandibular
- Mental nerve
- Buccal nerve
- Auriculotemporal nerve

Table 1.1 Branches of cranial nerve V (trigeminal nerve)

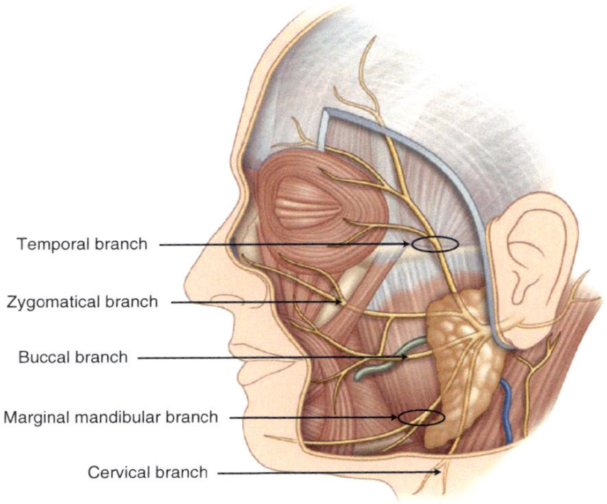

Figure 1.5 Branches of the facial nerve (*circles* indicate areas at greatest risk for injury)

- Temporal branch
- Zygomatical branch
- Buccal branch
- Marginal mandibular branch
- Cervical branch

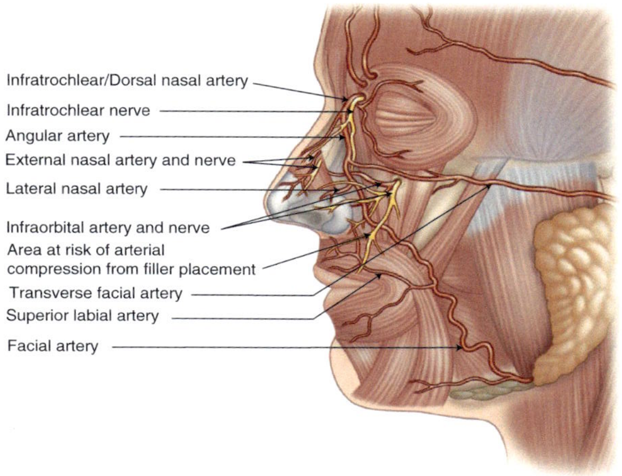

Section A Surgical Anatomy

Infratrochlear/Dorsal nasal artery
Infratrochlear nerve
Angular artery
External nasal artery and nerve
Lateral nasal artery
Infraorbital artery and nerve
Area at risk of arterial compression from filler placement
Transverse facial artery
Superior labial artery
Facial artery

Figure 1.6 Vascular supply to the face. *Source:* Reprint from Nouri, K. Complications in dermatologic surgery. Philadelphia, PA: Mosby Elsevier, 2008

6

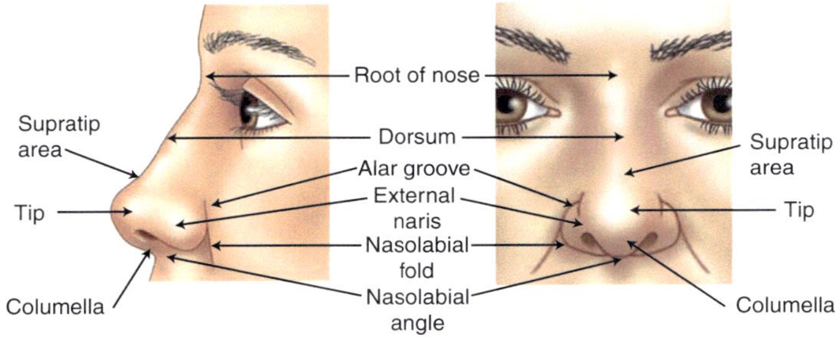

Section A Surgical Anatomy

Figure 1.7 Anatomy of the nose

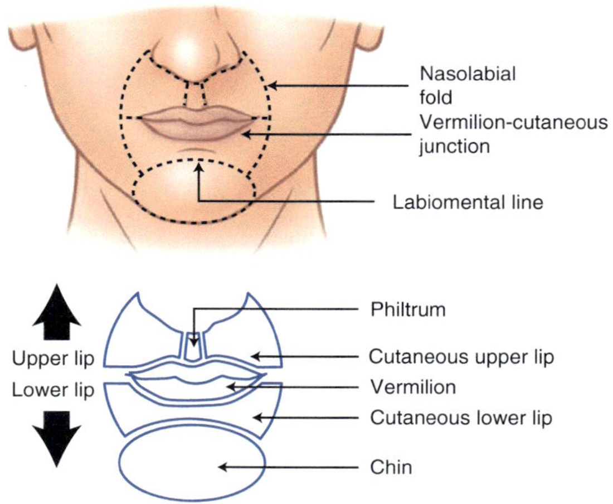

Section A Surgical Anatomy

- Nasolabial fold
- Vermilion-cutaneous junction
- Labiomental line

- Philtrum
- Cutaneous upper lip
- Vermilion
- Cutaneous lower lip
- Chin

Upper lip
Lower lip

Figure 1.8 Subunits of the face

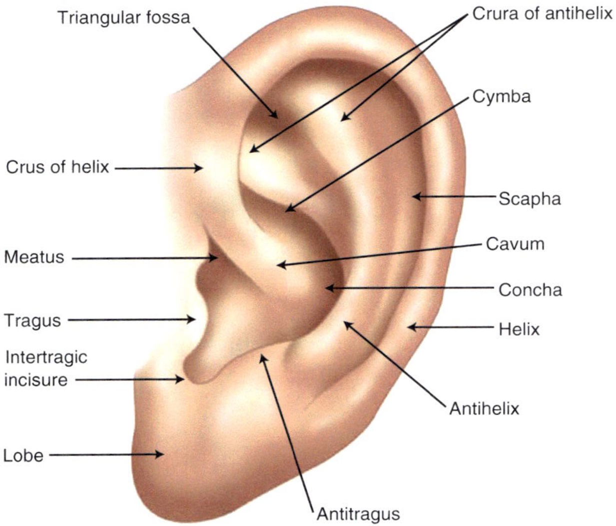

Section A Surgical Anatomy

Figure 1.9 Anatomy of the external ear

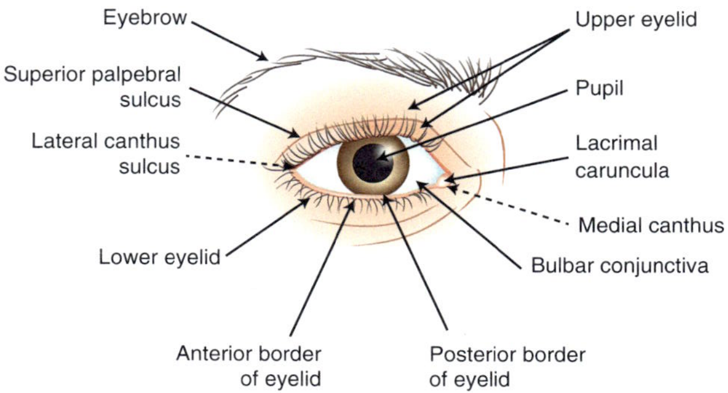

Section A Surgical Anatomy

Figure 1.10 Anatomy of the eye

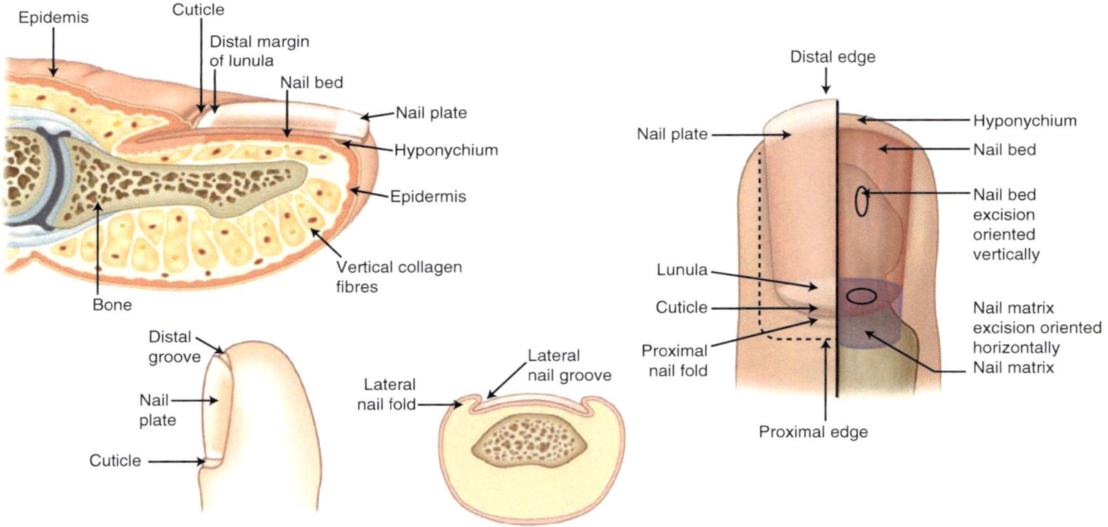

Section A Surgical Anatomy

Figure 1.11 Anatomy of the nail unit

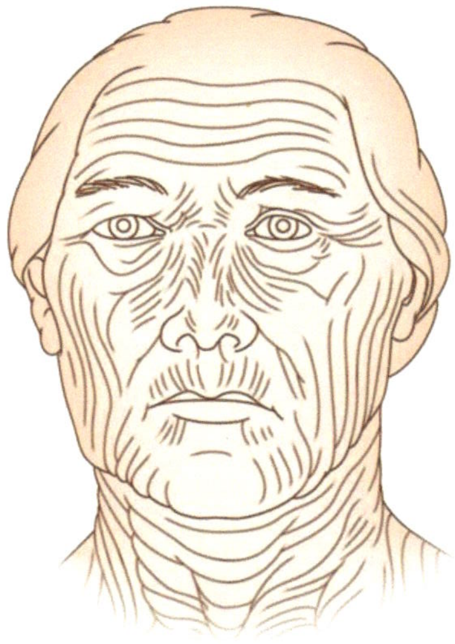

Section A **Surgical Anatomy**

Figure 1.12 Skin tension lines (*face*): for planning optimal incisions to minimize scarring

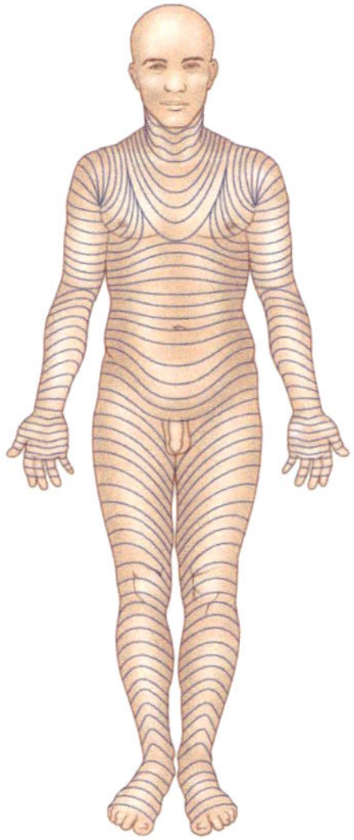

Section A   **Surgical Anatomy**

Figure 1.13 Skin tension lines (anterior)

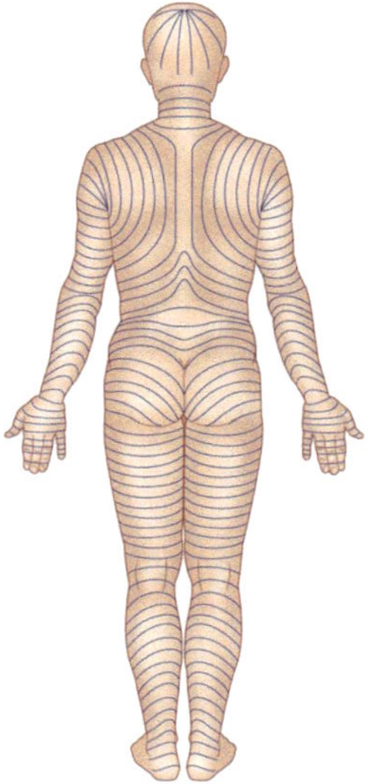

Section A Surgical Anatomy

Figure 1.14 Skin tension lines (posterior)

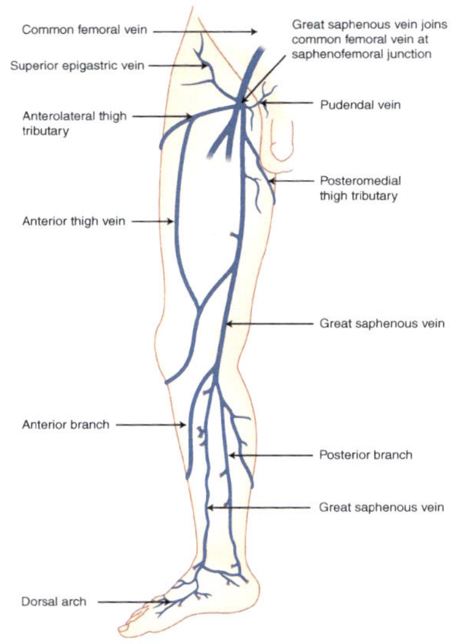

Section A   Surgical Anatomy

Figure 1.15 Great saphenous vein (GSV) and its tributaries

15

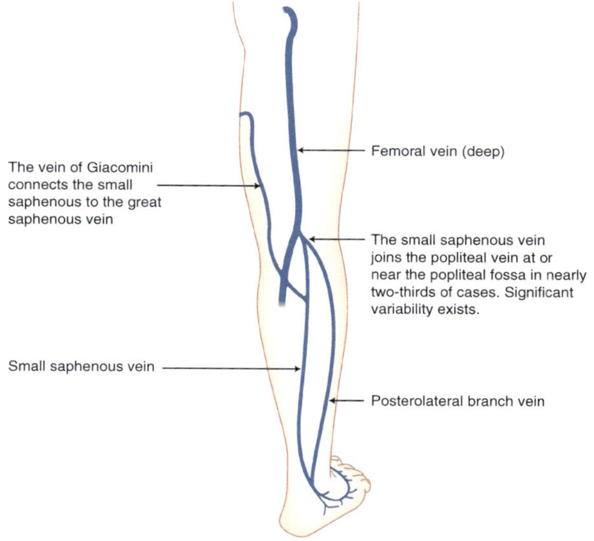

Section A Surgical Anatomy

Femoral vein (deep)

The small saphenous vein joins the popliteal vein at or near the popliteal fossa in nearly two-thirds of cases. Significant variability exists.

Posterolateral branch vein

The vein of Giacomini connects the small saphenous to the great saphenous vein

Small saphenous vein

Figure 1.16 Small saphenous vein (SSV) and its tributaries

Section B: Excisional and Non-excisional Surgery

Preoperative History

Medical history with particular attention to:

- Coronary artery disease
- Hypertension
- Arrhythmias
- Pacemaker or defibrillator
- Heart murmurs
- Artificial heart valves
- Prosthesis or shrapnel
- Bleeding or clotting disorders
- Hepatitis or HIV
- Keloids or hypertrophic scars
- Alcohol use
- Cigarette smoking
- Pregnancy (consider consultation with obstetrician)

Medications with particular attention to:

- Anticoagulants (recommendations on next page)
- Herbal and over the counter medications including but not limited to:
  - Vitamin E
  - Feverfew
  - Fish oil
  - Garlic
  - Ginger
  - Gingko biloba
  - Ginseng

Section B — Excisional and Non-excisional Surgery

  – Others: dong quai, licorice, devil's claw, and danshen have the same antithrombotic effect and should be discontinued 7–10 days preoperatively

• Recent use of oral retinoids (e.g., isotretinoin): may impair healing

• Immunosuppressants (e.g., TNF-inhibitors, cyclosporine, methotrexate, mycophenolate mofetil, and prednisone): may impair healing

• Medication allergies

Recommendations for management of anticoagulants:

• *Aspirin*: irreversibly inhibits platelet aggregation via acetylation of cyclooxygenase. One aspirin affects a platelet throughout its lifespan of 6–10 days. Medically indicated aspirin should not be stopped. However, if the patient can safely discontinue aspirin without a high risk for stroke or myocardial infarction, it should be withheld for 10 days before surgery and then possibly 5–7 days after surgery (after consultation with the patient's internist or cardiologist when appropriate). There may be a risk of rebound hypercoagulability with cessation.

• *Thienopyridines* (e.g., clopidogrel, ticlopidine): irreversibly inhibit platelet aggregation via inhibition of an ADP receptor on platelets. Normal platelet function returns 5–7 days

| Section B | **Excisional and Non-excisional Surgery** |

after discontinuing these medications. In patients on these drugs for cardiac or neurologic indications, it is generally not advisable to stop the drug.

- *Warfarin* (Coumadin): inhibits vitamin K dependent clotting factors and is commonly used in patients with a history of atrial fibrillation, DVT, and in patients with artificial heart valves. Dermatologic surgery can be safely performed without stopping warfarin as long as the INR ≤ 3. An INR should be checked within a week of planned surgery.

- *Dabigatran etexilate* (Pradaxa®): is an oral direct thrombin inhibitor used to reduce the risk of stroke and blood clots in patients with atrial fibrillation (not caused by heart valve abnormalities) and generally should be continued.

Note: The combination of two or more of these agents likely increases the risk of bleeding complications from surgery and temporary cessation of one of these agents after appropriate consultation with the cardiologist/internist/neurologist should be considered.

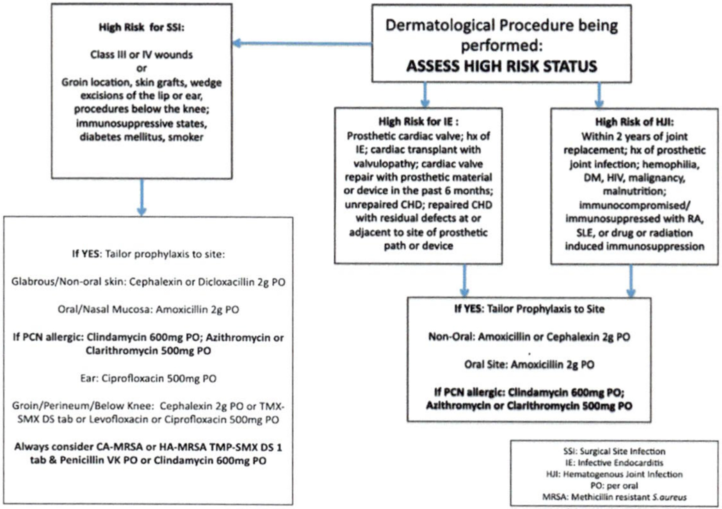

Section B Excisional and Non-excisional Surgery

High Risk for SSI:

Class III or IV wounds
or
Groin location, skin grafts, wedge excisions of the lip or ear, procedures below the knee; immunosuppressive states, diabetes mellitus, smoker

If YES: Tailor prophylaxis to site:

Glabrous/Non-oral skin: Cephalexin or Dicloxacillin 2g PO

Oral/Nasal Mucosa: Amoxicillin 2g PO

If PCN allergic: Clindamycin 600mg PO; Azithromycin or Clarithromycin 500mg PO

Ear: Ciprofloxacin 500mg PO

Groin/Perineum/Below Knee: Cephalexin 2g PO or TMX-SMX DS tab or Levofloxacin or Ciprofloxacin 500mg PO

Always consider CA-MRSA or HA-MRSA TMP-SMX DS 1 tab & Penicillin VK PO or Clindamycin 600mg PO

Dermatological Procedure being performed:
ASSESS HIGH RISK STATUS

High Risk for IE:

Prosthetic cardiac valve; hx of IE; cardiac transplant with valvulopathy; cardiac valve repair with prosthetic material or device in the past 6 months; unrepaired CHD; repaired CHD with residual defects at or adjacent to site of prosthetic path or device

High Risk of HJI:

Within 2 years of joint replacement; hx of prosthetic joint infection; hemophilia, DM, HIV, malignancy, malnutrition; immunocompromised/immunosuppressed with RA, SLE, or drug or radiation induced immunosuppression

If YES: Tailor Prophylaxis to Site

Non-Oral: Amoxicillin or Cephalexin 2g PO

Oral Site: Amoxicillin 2g PO

If PCN allergic: Clindamycin 600mg PO; Azithromycin or Clarithromycin 500mg PO

SSI: Surgical Site Infection
IE: Infective Endocarditis
HJI: Hematogenous Joint Infection
PO: per oral
MRSA: Methicillin resistant S.aureus

Figure 2.1 Guidelines for prophylactic and empiric antibiotics. Adapted from Rossi A, Mariwalla K. Prophylactic and empiric use of antibiotics in dermatologic surgery: a review of the literature and practical considerations. Dermatol Surg 2012;38:1898–1921

Section B Excisional and Non-excisional Surgery

Table 2.1 Commonly used prophylactic antibiotic agents for cutaneous surgery

Antibiotic	Spectrum of activity/notes
Dicloxacillin	*Staphylococcus* (methicillin sensitive), *Streptococcus*
Cephalosporins (e.g., Cephalexin)	Gram+ cocci, *E. coli*, *Klebsiella*, Proteus
Clindamycin, Erythromycin, Azithromycin	If PCN allergy (note: approximately 30% may be resistant to erythromycin)
Fluoroquinolones (e.g., Ciprofloxacin)	*Pseudomonas aeruginosa*
Vancomycin (intravenous)	Methicillin-resistant *Staph aureus* (MRSA), *Staph epidermidis*, Valve <60 days
Linezolid (po)	MRSA and vancomycin-resistant enterococcus, streptococcus (note: can cause thrombocytopenia)

An oral dose is usually given 1–2 h prior to surgery. If surgery is prolonged or delayed, a second dose may be given 6 h postoperatively

Section B Excisional and Non-excisional Surgery

Table 2.2 Antiseptic scrubs

Group	Spectrum	Onset	Sustained activity	Comments
Alcohol	Gram+	Fast	None	No killing of spores, antibacterial only, flammable (caution with electrocautery)
Iodine (Lugol's)	Gram+/−	Fast	None	May sensitize patient (contact dermatitis)
Povidone-iodine (betadine)	Gram+/−, fungi	Moderate	Up to 1 h	Absorbed through skin, must dry to be effective, mucosal absorption during pregnancy may be associated with fetal hypothyroidism
Hexachlorophene (pHisohex)	Gram+	Slow	Yes	Teratogen, not sporicidal
Chlorhexidine (hibiclens)	Gram+/−	Fast	Yes	Oculotoxicity and ototoxicity
Benzalkonium (Zephiran)	Gram+/−	Slow	None	

Note: shaving a preoperative site the night before surgery is associated with higher infection rates than with using a depilatory or not removing the hair at all. If hair must be removed, clipping the hair immediately before the procedure is preferable

Section B Excisional and Non-excisional Surgery

Table 2.3 Local anesthetics

Generic name/trade name	Duration	Onset	Uses	Special considerations	Maximum dosage with epi[a] (1:100,000)
Amides					
Lidocaine (Xylocaine®)	1–2 h with epinephrine	Rapid	Most local infiltration	May cause CNS and cardiac toxicity, pregnancy class B (without epi)	7 mg/kg
Mepivacaine (Carbocaine®)	1–2 h with epinephrine	3–20 min	Most local infiltration and nerve blocks		7 mg/kg
Bupivacaine (Marcaine®)	12–36 h	5–8 min	Nerve blocks and long procedures	Very prolonged effect, good for post-op pain	

(continued)

Section B Excisional and Non-excisional Surgery

Table 2.3 (continued)

Generic name/trade name	Duration	Onset	Uses	Special considerations	Maximum dosage with epi[a] (1:100,000)
Esters					
Procaine (Novocaine®)	30–60 min	2–5 min	Dental procedures	Short duration; allergic reactions; and cross-reacts with topical anesthetics, hair dyes, sunscreens, and sulfur derivatives	15 mg/kg
Tetracaine (Pontocaine®)	4–6 h	15–45 min	Topical (cornea, conjunctiva)	Slow onset, long duration	

[a]Epinephrine prolongs anesthesia and decreased the risk of systemic anesthetic toxicity due to decreased absorption via vasoconstriction. Also decreases bleeding via vasoconstriction

Section B Excisional and Non-excisional Surgery

Anesthetics: Key Facts

- Two main classes: Amides and Esters
- Esters can cause allergic reaction due to PABA (an ester intermediate metabolite) which cross-reacts with paraphenylenediamine (PPD), sulfonamides, and other ester anesthetics
- Esters should not be used in patients with pseudocholinesterase deficiency
- Three portions of the chemical structure:
  1. Aromatic: responsible for onset of activity
  2. Intermediate (middle) chain: determines class (amide vs. ester)
  3. Amine: determines duration of action
- Bupivacaine has the longest duration of action
- Tetracaine is the most potent ester
- Cocaine is the most vasoconstrictive ester
- Lidocaine Pearls:
  1. 1 % lidocaine = 10 mg/mL
  2. Pregnancy class B (without epinephrine)
  3. Lidocaine toxicity: first sign is lightheadedness/circumoral paresthesia/metallic taste→tinnitus/slurred speech/tremor/confusion→seizure/cardiopulmonary depression/death/coma
  4. Recommended maximum dosage with epinephrine = 7 mg/kg (500 mg in 70 kg

Section B Excisional and Non-excisional Surgery

person), without epinephrine (plain) 4.5 mg/kg (300 mg total in 70 kg person), Tumescent lidocaine 45–55 mg/kg (see Table 2.4/page 27)
- Digital tourniquets can be left on for 10–15 min
- Local anesthetics mechanism of action: blocking sodium influx
- Patient loses the following in this order: sense of temperature, pain, touch, pressure, vibration, proprioception, and motor function
- Epinephrine toxicity manifested by tremor, increased heart rate, diaphoresis, palpitations, headache, increased blood pressure, and chest pain (if hypotension consider vasovagal reaction rather than toxicity)
- Epinephrine drug contraindications: MAOIs, tricyclic antidepressants, phenothiazines, propranolol, amphetamines, and digitalis
- Epinephrine contraindications: peripheral vascular disease, acute angle glaucoma, severe hyperthyroidism, unstable mental status, pregnancy, severe hypertension or cardiovascular disease
- Other options for injectable anesthesia include promethazine (Phenergan), diphenhydramine (Benadryl), and normal saline
- Topical anesthesia:
  1. EMLA (eutectic mixture of 2.5 % lidocaine, 2.5 % prilocaine) under occlusion—Note: risk of methehemoglobinemia with prilocaine in infants
  2. LMX (4 or 5 % lidocaine)

Section B Excisional and Non-excisional Surgery

Table 2.4 Tumescent anesthesia solution

Agent	Amount (cc)	Final concentration
Normal saline (0.9 %)	1,000	
Lidocaine 1 %	50	0.1 %
Epinephrine 1:1,000	1	1:1,000,000
Bicarbonate 8.4 %	10	

Notes
[a]Maximum safe dose of lidocaine: 45–55 mg/kg
[b]Local anesthesia persists for up to 24 h after tumescent liposuction (peak plasma levels 4–14 h)

Section B Excisional and Non-excisional Surgery

Table 2.5 Electrosurgery

Modality	Terminal[a]	Voltage[b]	Amperage[c]	Comments
Electrofulgaration	1	Very high	Very low	Sparks emanate from electrode which does not touch the skin, most superficial damage
Electrodessication	1	High	Low	Electrode touches the tissue, superficial destruction (avascular lesions)
Electrocoagulation	2	Low	High	Deeper penetration and better hemostasis than electrodessication
Electrosection	2	Low	High	Vaporizes tissues with little heat spread, minimal peripheral tissue damage

(continued)

Section B Excisional and Non-excisional Surgery

Table 2.5 (continued)

Modality	Terminal[a]	Voltage[b]	Amperage[c]	Comments
Electrocautery	1	N/A	N/A	Red, hot tip (high resistance metal tip). Works in bloody fields and nonconductive surfaces. No current passes through patient—**safest to use with ICD**[d]
Galvanic current	1	Low	Low	Direct current, used for electrolysis and iontophoresis

[a] Terminal: 1 terminal (aka monopolar): one active electrode, no grounding; 2 terminals (aka bipolar): one active electrode, one grounding electrode (place grounding pad close to surgery site and aware from ICD)
[b] Voltage: electric potential difference between the terminal and the skin
[c] Amperage reflects the flow of electric current
[d] ICD (implantable cardiac device)

Section B: Excisional and Non-excisional Surgery

Cryosurgery

Defined: Targeted tissue destruction via necrosis induced by subzero temperatures

Agent	Boiling point (°C)
Liquid nitrogen	–195.6
Nitrous oxide	–89.5
Dry ice (CO_2)	–78.5
Freon	–40.8 to –3.8
Ethyl chloride	13.1

Section B Excisional and Non-excisional Surgery

Cell type	Temperature required (°C)
Melanocyte necrosis[a]	−5
Keratinocyte necrosis	−25
Benign lesion treatment	−25
Skin cancer treatment	−50

[a]Therefore risk of hypopigmentation with cryosurgery

Section B Excisional and Non-excisional Surgery

Table 2.6 Recommended surgical margins

Melanoma (based on breslow depth)[a]	Margin size	Comments
In situ	0.5 cm[b]	Lentigo maligna on the face consider 0.7–1 cm margins vs. staged excision vs. Mohs surgery (with immunostains)
≤1 mm	1 cm	Consider sentinel lymph node biopsy in <1 mm melanoma if ulceration or mitotic rate $\geq 1 \text{ mm}^{-2}$
1.01–2 mm	1–2 cm	
>2 mm	2 cm+	
Squamous cell carcinoma		
Low risk	3–4 mm	
High risk[c]	6 mm	Consider Mohs surgery

(continued)

Section B Excisional and Non-excisional Surgery

Table 2.6 (continued)

Melanoma (based on breslow depth)[a]	Margin size	Comments
Basal cell carcinoma		
<2 cm	3–4 mm	
≥2 cm	6 mm	Consider Mohs surgery

[a]Sladden MJ, et al. Surgical excision margins for primary cutaneous melanoma. Cochrane Database Syst Rev. 2009;(4):CD004855

[b]Recent data suggests that current recommended margins are inadequate, with only 86 % of melanoma in-situ's completely excised with 6 mm margins, whereas 9 mm margins remove 98.9 % of melanoma in-situ's. Kunishige JH. et al. Surgical margins for melanoma in situ. J Am Acad Dermatol. 2012;66(3):438–44

[c]High-risk cutaneous SCC defined by the following: poor differentiation, perineural invasion, tumor diameter ≥2 cm, and invasion beyond subcutaneous fat. Jambusaria-Pahlajani A, et al. Evaluation of AJCC tumor staging for cutaneous squamous cell carcinoma and a proposed alternative tumor staging system. JAMA Dermatol. 2013;16:1–9

Section B Excisional and Non-excisional Surgery

Table 2.7 Melanoma staging

Melanoma TNM classification

T classification	Thickness	Ulceration status/mitoses
Tis	N/A	N/A
T1	≤1.0 mm	a: Without ulceration and mitosis <1 mm^{-2}
		b: With ulceration or mitoses ≥1 mm^{-2}
T2	1.01–2.0 mm	a: Without ulceration
		b: With ulceration
T3	2.01–4.0 mm	a: Without ulceration
		b: With ulceration

(continued)

Section B Excisional and Non-excisional Surgery

Table 2.7 (continued)

Melanoma TNM classification

T4	>4.0 mm	a: Without ulceration
		b: With ulceration
N classification	Number of metastatic nodes	Nodal metastatic mass
N0	0	N/A
N1	1 node	a: Micrometastasis[a]
		b: Macrometastasis[b]
N2	2–3 nodes	a: Micrometastasis[a]
		b: Macrometastasis[b]
		c: In-transit met(s)/satellite(s)[c] without metastatic node(s)

(continued)

Section B Excisional and Non-excisional Surgery

Table 2.7 (continued)

Melanoma TNM classification

N3	4 or more metastatic nodes, matted nodes, or in-transit met(s)/satellite(s)[c] with metastatic node(s)	

M classification	Site	Serum lactate dehydrogenase
M0	No distant metastases	N/A
M1a	Distant skin, subcutaneous or nodal metastases	Normal
M1b	Lung metastases	Normal

(continued)

Section B Excisional and Non-excisional Surgery

Table 2.7 (continued)

Melanoma TNM classification

		Normal
M1c	All other visceral metastases	
	Any distant metastasis	Elevated

Melanoma TNM classification. For defining T1 melanomas Clark level of invasion is used as default criterion only if mitotic rate cannot be determined. Histologic evaluation of lymph nodes must include at least one immunohistochemical marker (e.g., HMB45, Melan-A/MART-1)

Adapted from Balch CM, Gershenwald JE, Soong SJ, et al. Final version of 2009 AJCC melanoma staging and classification. J Clin Oncol. 2009;27: 6199–6206

NA not applicable

[a]Micrometastases are diagnosed after sentinel or elective lymphadenectomy

[b]Macrometastases are defined as clinically detectable nodal metastases confirmed by therapeutic lymphadenectomy or when nodal metastasis exhibits gross extracapsular extension

[c]In-transit metastases are >2 cm from the primary tumor but not beyond the regional lymph nodes, while satellite lesions are within 2 cm of the primary

Section B: Excisional and Non-excisional Surgery

Main Indications for Mohs Micrographic Surgery

- Non-melanoma skin cancer (BCC/SCC) in high-risk anatomic locations (periorbital, perinasal, periauricular, perioral, and hair-bearing scalp), or tissue sparing location (genitals, digits)
- Poorly defined tumors
- Recurrent tumors
- Aggressive histology (morpheaform, micronodular and infiltrating BCCs, SCC with poor differentiation, and infiltrative or spindle cell SCC)
- Perineural invasion
- Dermatofibrosarcoma protuberans, atypical fibroxanthoma, microcystic adnexal carcinoma, merkel cell carcinoma, extramammary paget's disease, and sebaceous carcinoma
- Tumors >2 cm in diameter
- Previous history of radiation treatment at site of malignancy
- Basal cell nevus syndrome, Xeroderma Pigmentosum
- Immunocompromised patients

Section B: Excisional and Non-excisional Surgery

Mohs Micrographic Surgery Procedure

- Disc excision of tumor with 1–2 mm margin with scalpel blade beveled at approximately 45° angle
- Tumor orientation is maintained and mapped
- Frozen sections prepared via sectioning in horizontal planes (vs. traditional breadloafing for permanent sections)
- Peripheral and deep margins examined by Mohs surgeon
- Process repeated until free margins obtained and closure vs. secondary intention healing

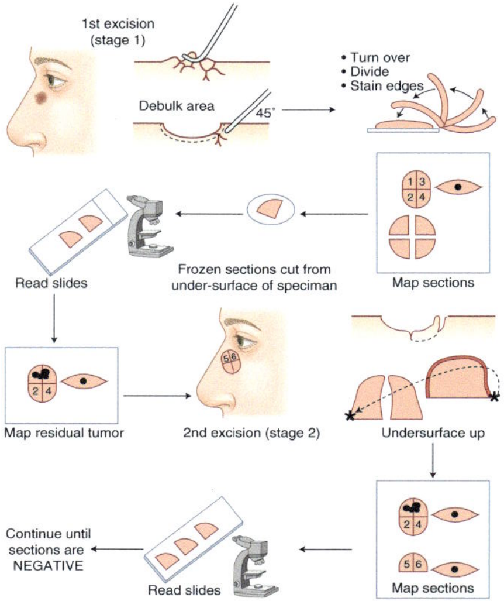

Section B: Excisional and Non-excisional Surgery

Figure 2.2 Mohs micrographic surgery. *Source:* Wolff K, Goldsmith LA, Katz SI, Gilchrest BA, Paller AS, Leffell DJ: *Fitzpatrick's Dermatology in General Medicine*, 7th Edition: http://accessmedicine.com. Copyright © The McGraw-Hill Companies, Inc. All rights reserved

Section B Excisional and Non-excisional Surgery

Elliptical Fusiform Excision

When/Where
Simple, basic excision, or an excisional biopsy performed on any part of the body.

How
The excision should have a length-to-width ratio of approximately 3:1 (Figure 2.3). Make the apical angles 30°. Such excisions should be placed parallel to relaxed skin tension lines whenever possible so that in time the scar will settle to resemble these preexisting lines.

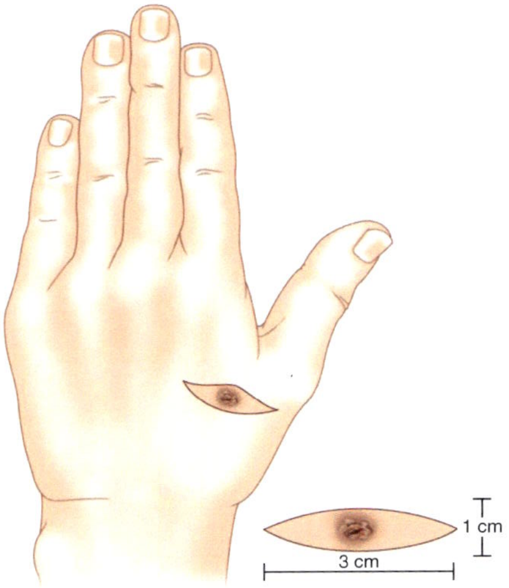

Figure 2.3 Elliptical fusiform excision

Section B Excisional and Non-excisional Surgery

Placement of Incisions and Excisions on the Face

When/Where
Incisions and Excisions on the face.

How
Ideally, all incisions should be oriented within or parallel to "lines of expression." Figure 2.4 shows suggested placement of excisions on the face based on common relaxed skin tension lines.

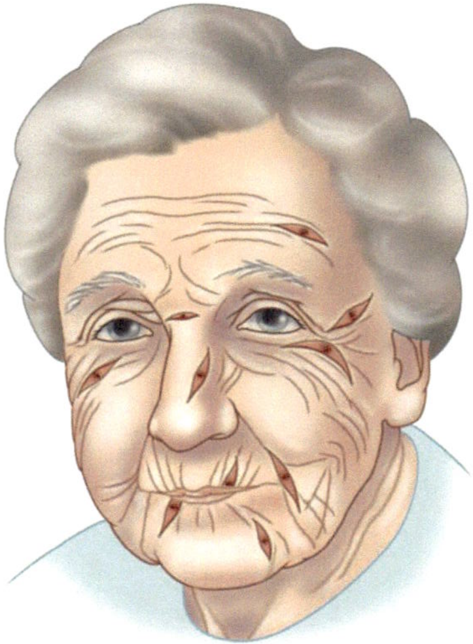

Figure 2.4 Placement of incisions and excisions on the face

Section B   Excisional and Non-excisional Surgery

Simple Interrupted Stitch

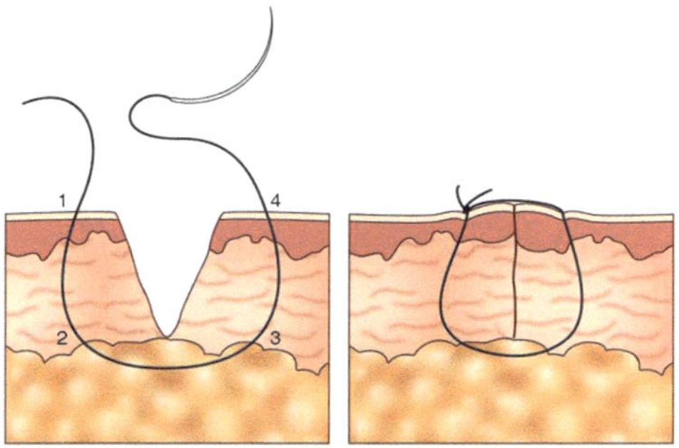

Figure 2.5 Simple interrupted stitch: the needle penetrates the epidermis (1) and is rotated slightly outward through the dermis and subcutaneous tissue in certain wounds (2). The needle then crosses the wound, looping a substantial portion of dermis and possibly subcutaneous tissue before being redirected upwards (3). The needle then exits the epidermis where the suture is then tied (4)

| Section B | **Excisional and Non-excisional Surgery** |

Buried Vertical Mattress Stitch

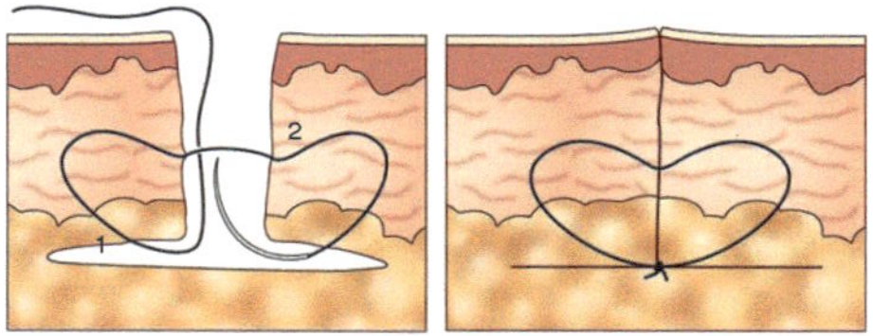

Figure 2.6 Buried vertical mattress stitch for deep dermal tissue approximation and eversion (1: place the curved needle in the subcutaneous tissue and make an arc upwards toward the superficial dermis, continuing the arc and exiting through the mid-dermis, then 2: this step is repeated on the opposite side entering through the mid-portion of the dermis, making an upward arc toward the upper reticular dermis, and continue the curve downward to exit the subcutaneous surface)

Section B Excisional and Non-excisional Surgery

Cutaneous Vertical Mattress Stitch

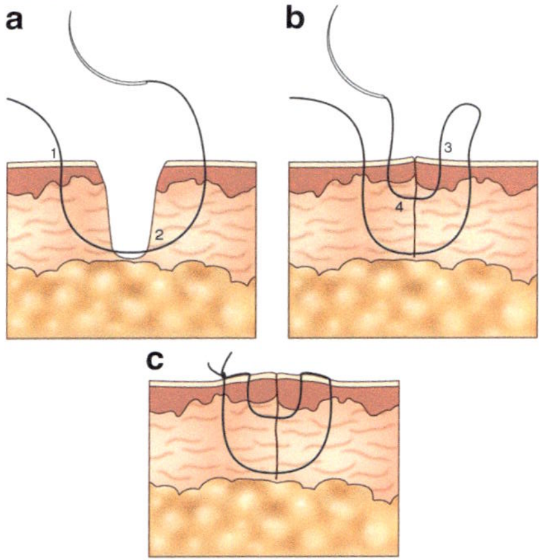

Figure 2.7 Vertical mattress stitch: (**a**) the needle is placed 5–10 mm from the wound edge, and a simple interrupted suture is placed (1, 2). (**b**) The needle is redirected back across the wound more superficially (3), penetrating the skin edge 2–4 mm from the wound on both sides (4). (**c**) Final appearance of this suture after tying

45

| Section B | Excisional and Non-excisional Surgery |

Horizontal Mattress Stitch

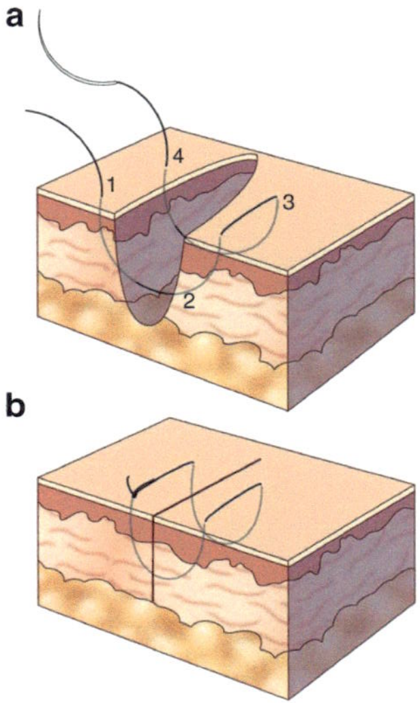

Figure 2.8 (a, b) Horizontal mattress stitch

| Section B | **Excisional and Non-excisional Surgery** |

Running Subcuticular Stitch

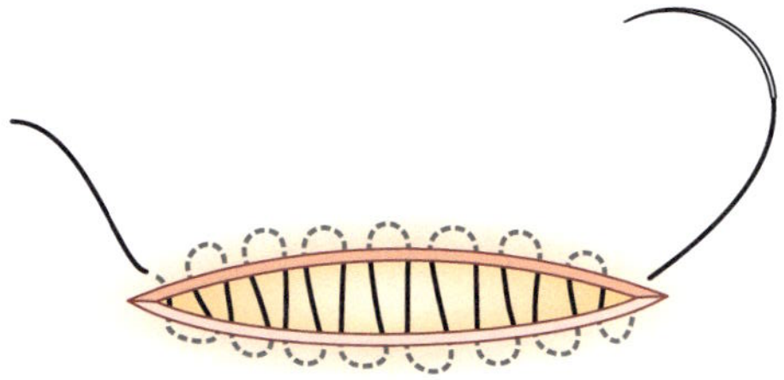

Figure 2.9 Running subcuticular/intradermal stitch: begin by either placing the needle from the external skin down into the epidermis and leaving the free end of the suture exposed (as with polyprolene) or by placing a buried vertical stitch at one end of the defect, cutting only the free suture tail. Then introduce the needle into the adjacent portion of the dermis of one side of the wound and advance the needle horizontally towards the other apex, exiting at the same plane. Then enter the needle into the dermis of the opposite side of the wound, just behind the point of needle exit. Continue to advance the needle intradermally, alternating sides until eventually exiting through the epidermis at the other apex of the wound

Section B   **Excisional and Non-excisional Surgery**

Pulley Stitch

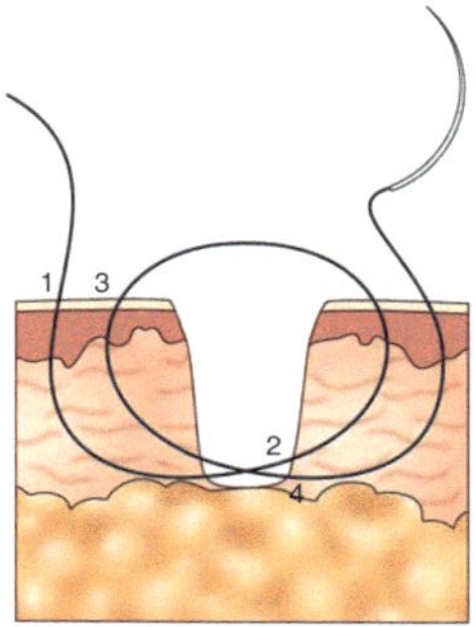

Figure 2.10 Pulley stitch (epidermal): for closure of wounds under tension. *Numbers* indicate points of entry

Section B Excisional and Non-excisional Surgery

Three Point Suture (aka Tip stitch)

When/Where
Where two cut surfaces come together that are not in a straight line. It is useful when suturing the tip of a pointed flap (this is known as a three-point suture, tip-stitch, or half- buried horizontal mattress).

How
The suture begins in the skin surface, penetrates to the level of the mid-dermis, emerges through the tip area, reenters the other side of the wound at the same mid-dermis level, and exits through the skin.

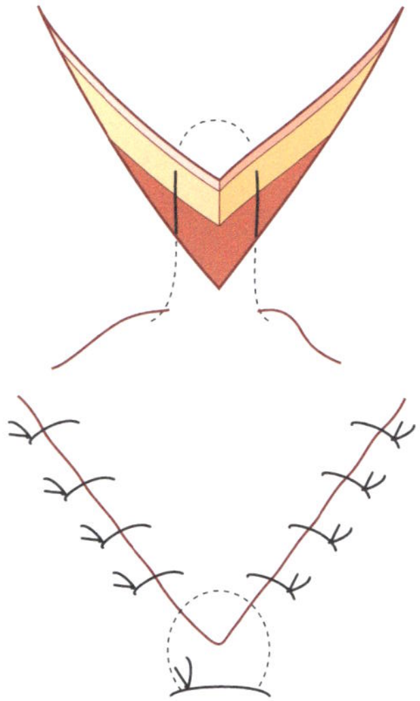

Figure 2.11 Three-point stitch (AKA tip stitch)

| Section B | **Excisional and Non-excisional Surgery** |

"Dog Ear" Repair

When/Where

Where there is excess of bulging skin at some point of a wound closure, which usually results when closure involves inadequate length-to-width ratio or an elliptical excision with sides of unequal length.

How

The simplest method is to elongate the excision line, which gives a greater ratio to the length–diameter proportion. Another method utilizes a skin hook placed in the apex of the fold and pulled to one side. One side is incised with a scalpel. This piece of tissue is then pulled to the opposite side of the wound and also incised with a scalpel. Sutures are then placed accordingly.

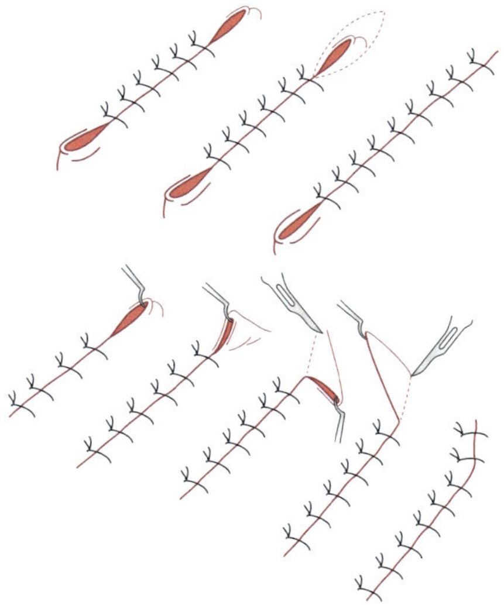

Figure 2.12 Repair of dog ears

Section B Excisional and Non-excisional Surgery

"Leashing" of Dog Ears

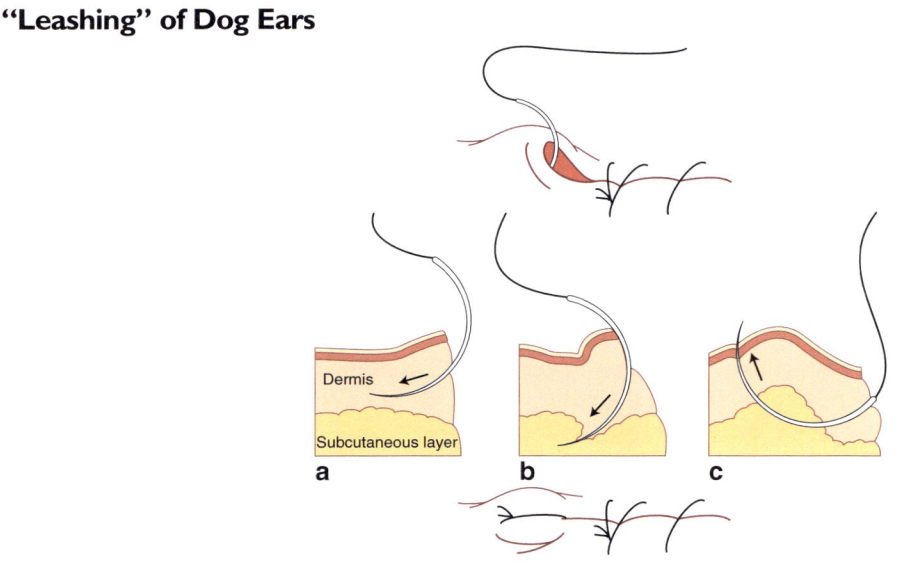

Figure 2.13 (continued)

Section B Excisional and Non-excisional Surgery

Figure 2.13 "Leashing" the dog ear after completely closing a wound with cutaneous sutures, a needle is inserted into the end of the suture line in the intradermal plane and in the direction of the "dog ear" (*top panel*, and **a**). The needle is advanced intradermally for approximately one third of the length of the needle parallel to the epidermis (*middle panel*, **a**). The needle is then directed downward until it penetrates the subcutaneous tissue (*middle panel*, **b**). The needle is then advanced a few millimeters forward in the superficial subcutaneous plane and is then directed upward through the dermis and epidermis (*middle panel*, **c**). The suture is then tied thereby "leashing" the "dog ear" by pulling it level with the suture line

Section B: Excisional and Non-excisional Surgery

Table 2.8 Absorbable sutures

Suture	Origin	Filament	Absorption	Reactivity	Tensile strength	Degradation
Plain gut	Animal collagen	Twisted	60–70 days	High	Poor	Proteolysis
Chromic gut	Animal collagen	Twisted	80 days	Moderate	Poor	Proteolysis
Vicryl (polyglactin 910)	Copolymer	Braided	80 days	Low	Good	Hydrolysis
Dexon (polyglycolic acid)	Homopolymer of glycolic acid	Braided	90 days	Low	Good	Hydrolysis

(continued)

Section B Excisional and Non-excisional Surgery

Table 2.8 (continued)

Suture	Origin	Filament	Absorption	Reactivity	Tensile strength	Degradation
PDS (polydioxanone)	Polyester polymer	Monofilament	180 days	Low	Greatest	Hydrolysis
Maxon (glycolic acid, polyglyconate)	Glycolic acid Trimethylene carbonate	Monofilament	180 days	Low	Great	Hydrolysis
Monocryl (polyglecaprone-25)	Copolymer of glycolide and epsilon-caprolactone	Monofilament	91–119 days	Low	Great	Hydrolysis

Section B: Excisional and Non-excisional Surgery

Table 2.9 Nonabsorbable sutures

Suture	Origin	Filament	Reactivity	Tensile strength	Uses
Silk	Silk	Braided or twisted	High	None at 1 year	Mucosal surfaces
Ethilon	Nylon	Monofilament	Low	High	Cutaneous, vessels
Dermalon	Nylon	Monofilament	Low	High	Cutaneous, vessels
Prolene	Polypropylene	Monofilament	Least	High	Running subcuticular (intradermal)
Mersilene	Polyester	Braided	Low	High	Cutaneous, knots well, cutaneous

Section B Excisional and Non-excisional Surgery

Table 2.10 Topical antimicrobial agents

Name	Components	Spectrum	Comments
Gentamycin		Gram−	Resistance
Neomycin		Gram−	No pseudomonas, yes proteus
Polymixin B		Gram−	Yes pseudomonas, no proteus
Bacitracin		Staph, strep	Risk of anaphylaxis (open wounds), allergic contact dermatitis
Neosporin	Neomycin/Bacitracin/Polymixin B	Broad	Risk of sensitization, co-sensitivity between neomycin and bacitracin (allergic contact dermatitis)
Polysporin	Bacitracin/Polymixin B	Broad	Risk of sensitization, allergic contact dermatitis

(continued)

Section B Excisional and Non-excisional Surgery

Table 2.10 (continued)

Name	Components	Spectrum	Comments
Bactroban	Mupirocin	Gram+	Kills b-lactamase + organisms
Silvadene	Silver sulfadiazine	Broad including yeast	Caution: sulfonamide hypersensitivity or G6PD deficiency
Dakin's	Sodium hypochlorite (bleach)		Not recommended for open wounds due to cytotoxicity
Vinegar	Acetic acid	Pseudomonas	

Section B — Excisional and Non-excisional Surgery

Table 2.11 Wound dressing

Type	Brand name	Characteristics	Purpose	Indications
Polyurethane films	Op-site, Tegaderm, Bioocclusive	Transparent thin semipermeable sheet	Allows air exchange but not fluid loss; promotes re-epithelialization; No absorption of wound drainage	Lacerations, abrasions
Hydrocolloids	Duoderm, Comfeel	Opaque sheet	Debrides wounds, stimulates granulation tissue of open wounds, and absorbs wound drainage	Chronic wound, protects injured surface, and moist or dry wound
Hydrogel	Vigilon, Nu-gel	Semitransparent gel	Absorbs wound drainage	Moist wound
Polyurethane foams	Synthoderm, Epiloch	Opaque, sponge-like	Compresses wound, no absorption of wound drainage	Compresses chronic leg wounds
Interface protector	Telfa pad, Vaseline gauze	Sheet or pad	Covers without improving healing	Covers without sticking

Section B Excisional and Non-excisional Surgery

Table 2.12 Surgical complications

Complication	Risk factors	Prevention and management
Bleeding and hematoma formation	Anticoagulant medications, hereditary bleeding disorders, larger procedures (flaps), and removal of space occupying lesions	Stop unnecessary anticoagulant medications (see recommendations section); adequate intraoperative hemostasis; and adequate pressure dressing Evacuate hematoma (remove sutures)
Damage to nerves or vital organs	Surgery in a high-risk location	Careful attention to local tissue anatomy (see Figure X Facial N diagram)
Anesthetic side effects	Cardiovascular disease	Limit total dose of anesthetics and epinephrine, avoid intravascular injection

(continued)

Section B Excisional and Non-excisional Surgery

Table 2.12 (continued)

Complication	Risk factors	Prevention and management
Electrosurgery complications	Pacemakers and defibrillators	Place grounding plate away from the ICD with bipolar devices Consult a cardiologist for defibrillators. Use short bursts to minimize electromagnetic interference
Contact dermatitis	Bacitracin, neomycin irritation from dressings	Identify and discontinue the offending agent
Infection	Diabetes, immunocompromised patients, prolonged procedures, breach of oral mucosa, surgery below the knee, TNF-inhibitors (or other immunosuppressant therapy), and surgery on inflamed skin	Sterile technique, antibiotics, wound culture, and wound care

(continued)

Section B Excisional and Non-excisional Surgery

Table 2.12 (continued)

Complication	Risk factors	Prevention and management
Chondritis	Surgery of the ear	NSAIDs, warm compresses
Wound dehiscence	High tension, heavy lifting, and hematomas	Allow secondary intention healing or resuture and prescribe antibiotics
Skin necrosis	Excessive tension, inadequate arterial supply	Wound care to allow secondary intention healing
Suture spitting	Long-lasting subcuticular sutures or superficial placement	Removal of spitting sutures
Suture track marks	Delayed removal of sutures, excessive tension	Timely removal of cuticular sutures; utilize running subcuticular sutures when possible

(continued)

Section B Excisional and Non-excisional Surgery

Table 2.12 (continued)

Complication	Risk factors	Prevention and management
Excessive granulation tissue	Secondary intention healing	Silver nitrate sticks, PDL
	Oral retinoid use	Topical and intralesional corticosteroids
Hyperpigmented scars	Dark-skinned patients, post-operative sun exposure	Topical hydroquinone, corticosteroids, retinoids, and pigment lasers
Hypopigmented scars	Dark-skinned patients	308-nm excimer laser, fractional ablation
Hypertrophic scars and keloids	Personal or family history of keloids; upper trunk location, excessive postoperative exertion or tension	Timely suture removal Intralesional corticosteroids, 5-FU, lasers, and topical silicone

Section B Excisional and Non-excisional Surgery

Table 2.13 Suture removal timetable

Site	Number of days
Face	4–7
Neck	7–10
Scalp	7–14
Thorax, arms	7–14
Legs, feet	14–21

Section B Excisional and Non-excisional Surgery

Commonly Used Surgical Instruments in Dermatologic Surgery

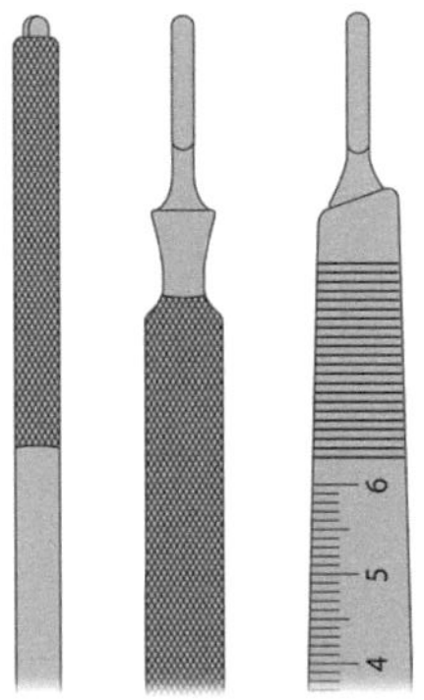

Figure 2.14 Scalpel handles: (*left to right*) the Beaver round knurled handle, the Bard-Parker round knurled #3 handle, and the Bard-Parker #3 standard handle

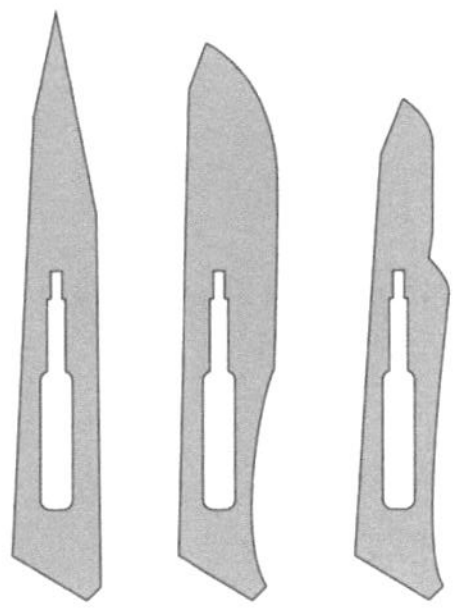

Section B Excisional and Non-excisional Surgery

Figure 2.15 Scalpel blades: the Bard-Parker #15 (*right*), #10 (*middle*), and #11 (*left*)

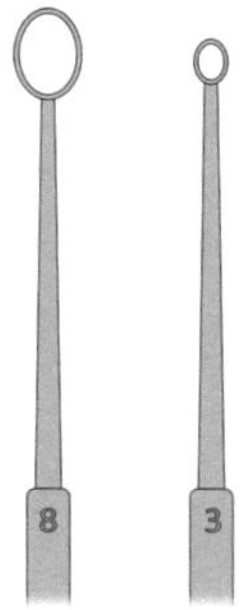

Section B Excisional and Non-excisional Surgery

Figure 2.16 Curettes: large (*left*) and small (*right*) variants with oval heads

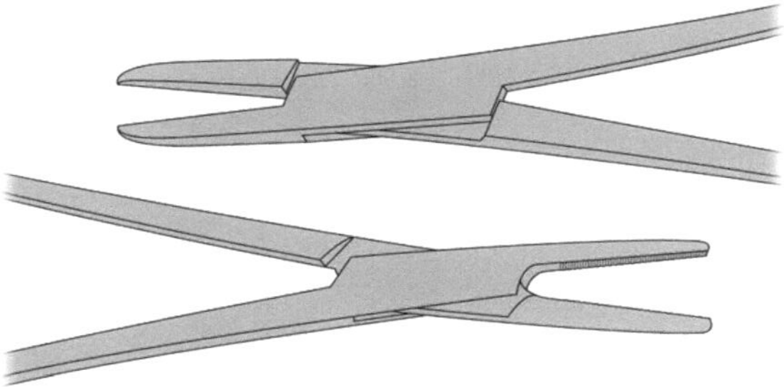

Section B

Excisional and Non-excisional Surgery

Figure 2.17 Needle holders: smooth (*top*) and fine-toothed (*bottom*) variants

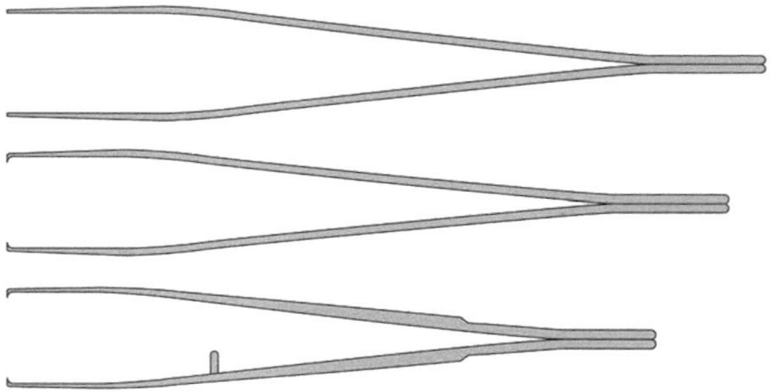

Section B | **Excisional and Non-excisional Surgery**

Figure 2.18 Adson Forceps: (*top to bottom*) heavy, smooth, straight forceps, heavy 1 × 2 toothed straight forceps, and delicate 1 × 2 toothed straight forceps

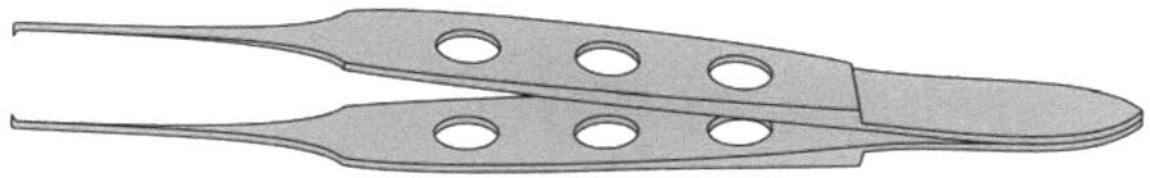

Section B: Excisional and Non-excisional Surgery

Figure 2.19 Bishop Harmon forceps

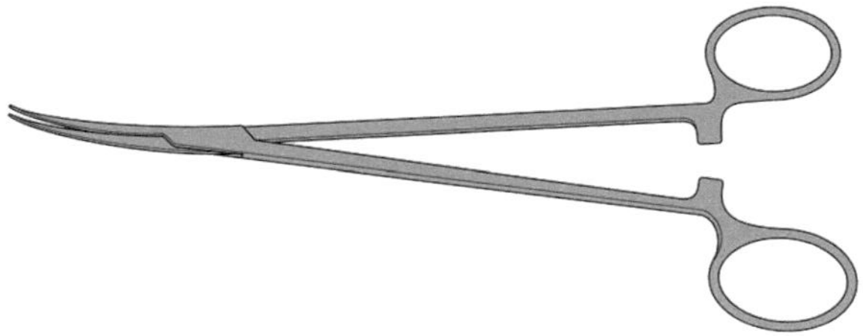

Section B: Excisional and Non-excisional Surgery

Figure 2.20 Jacobson hemostat forceps

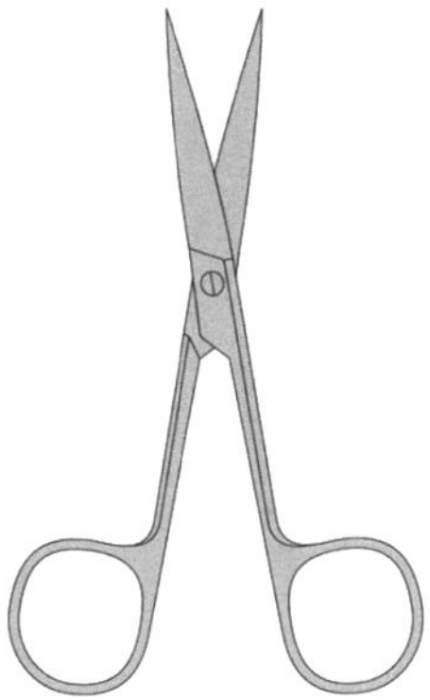

Section B Excisional and Non-excisional Surgery

Figure 2.21 Scissors: general operating scissors for suture cutting

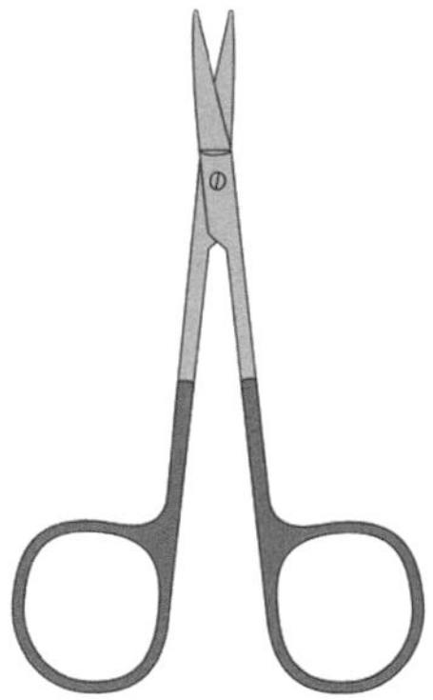

Section B: Excisional and Non-excisional Surgery

Figure 2.22 Curved metzenbaum scissor

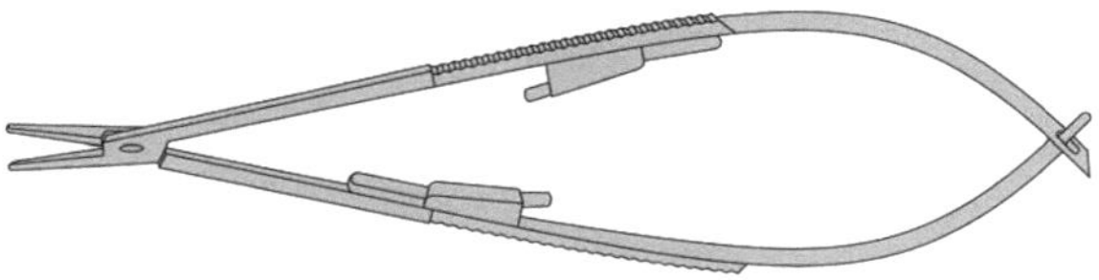

Section B: Excisional and Non-excisional Surgery

Figure 2.23 Castroviejo needle driver

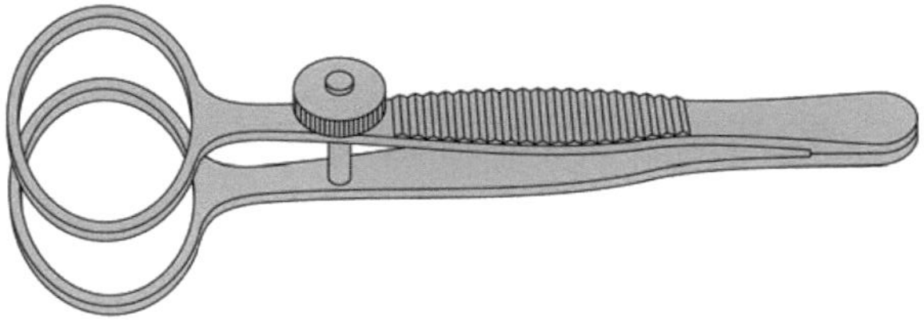

Section B: Excisional and Non-excisional Surgery

Figure 2.24 Chalazion clamp

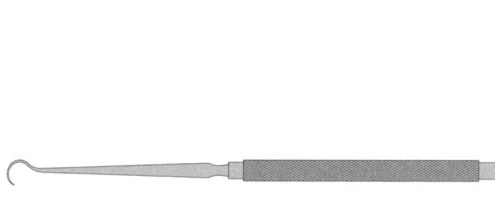

Section B: Excisional and Non-excisional Surgery

Figure 2.25 Skin hook

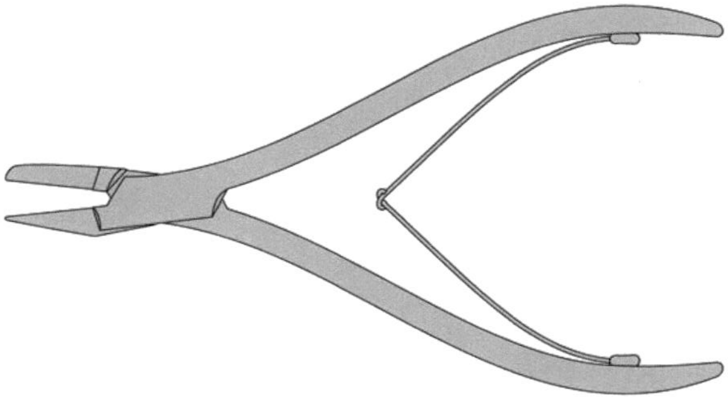

Section B | **Excisional and Non-excisional Surgery**

Figure 2.26 English nail splitter

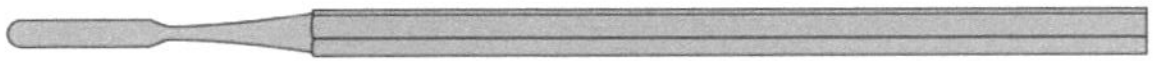

Section B: Excisional and Non-excisional Surgery

Figure 2.27 Nail elevator

Section C Advanced Repairs

Flap Overview

Classified Based on Primary Tissue Movement or Vascular Supply

Axial Flap: axial cutaneous flaps include a named artery within the flap's longitudinal axis, used to repair larger defects (commonly nasal defects). Examples include median and paramedian forehead flaps (supratrochlear A.), the dorsal nasal flap (angular A.), and the Abbe cross-lip flap (labial A.)

Random Pattern: geometrically designed surgical repair based on either deep or adjacent vascular pedicles without named arterial blood supply, the elevated portion of the flap is perfused by the highly anastomotic subdermal and dermal vascular network.

Interpolation: staged flap in which base of flaps pedicle is noncontiguous with surgical wound, can be axial (e.g., paramedian forehead flap, and Abbe cross-lip flap) or random pattern (e.g., melolabial). Division of the pedicle is typically done at approximately day 21 but varies with surgeon preference and type of repair.

Section C Advanced Repairs

Single Advancement Flap

When/Where

To cover a defect where adequate tissue on one side is available to slide over the defect to facilitate good closure. Especially useful in areas where the parallel lines of the flap will fit into normal wrinkle lines such as those on the forehead and eyebrow. Patients with good laxity of skin (e.g., the elderly) are suitable candidates.

How

Parallel lines are cut, tissue and flap are freed from their base and slid over the defect to join with adjacent tissue. Small Burow's triangles may be necessary to remove bulging at the base of the flap.

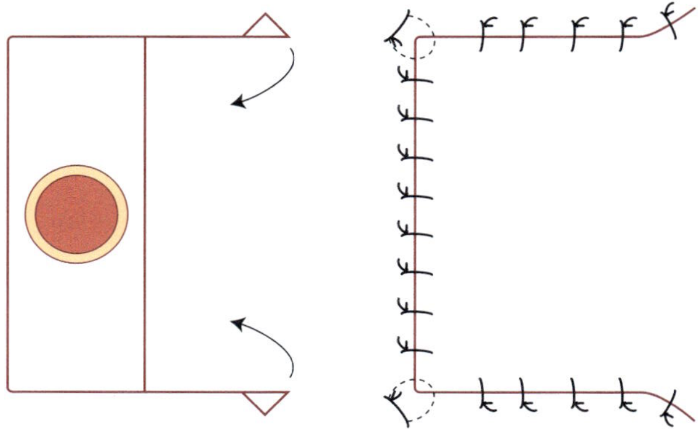

Figure 3.1 Single advancement flap

Section C Advanced Repairs

Bilateral Advancement Flap (H-Plasty)

When/Where

Where it is more judicious to slide tissue from both directions to achieve good closure. Frequently used on the scalp and the upper lip.

How

See "Single Advancement Flap" section

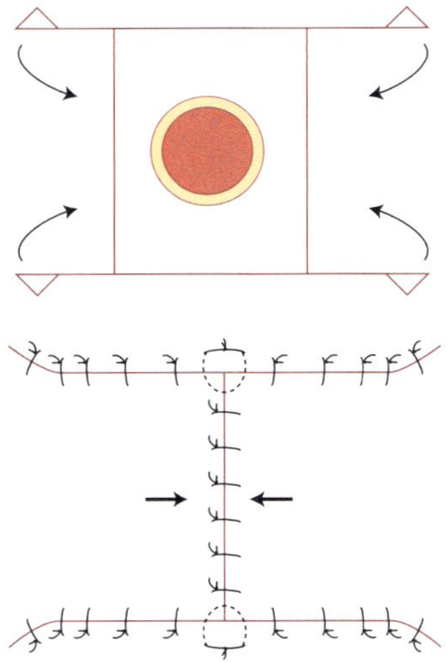

Figure 3.2 Bilateral advancement flap

Section C Advanced Repairs

Z-Plasty

When/Where
Mainly used to change the direction of a scar that is deforming (e.g., a long scar line) or to elongate a scar that is constricting (redirect tension vectors). Common sites for usage are the medial canthus, side of the face, and forehead.

How
Incise a Z-plasty using 60° angles; the limbs of the Z should be of equal length. The amount of tissue available on either side will determine how long the common limb of the Z (and thus, the size of the Z-plasty) can be.

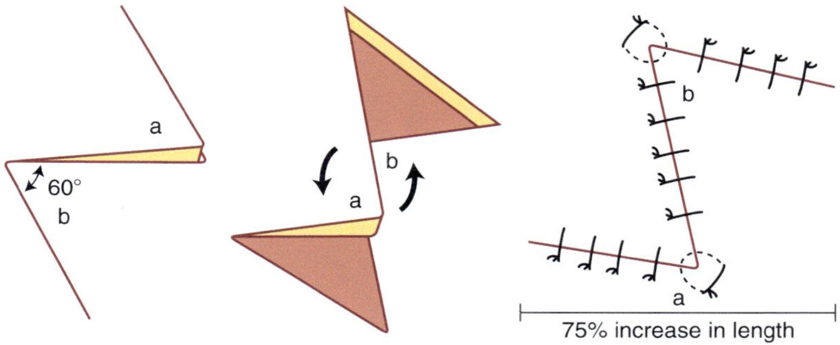

Figure 3.3 Z-plasty

| Section C | **Advanced Repairs** |

M-Plasty

When/Where

When it is desirable not to extend an ellipse into a nearby structure or to avoid cutting across relaxed skin tension lines (reduce scar length).

Figure 3.5 shows suggested placement sites on the face (e.g., eyebrow, outer canthus, nasolabial fold, and lips).

How

This excision makes use of 30° angles at the apices (Fig. 3.4). The amount of tissue saved is shown in the shaded area. Interrupted sutures and a three-point suture are used to close the wound.

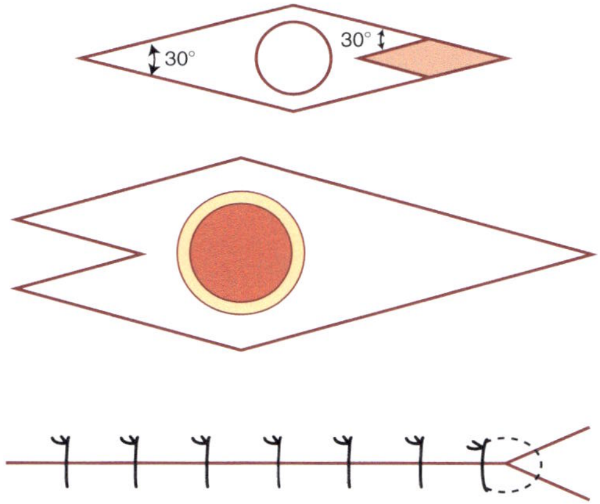

Figure 3.4 M-plasty

83

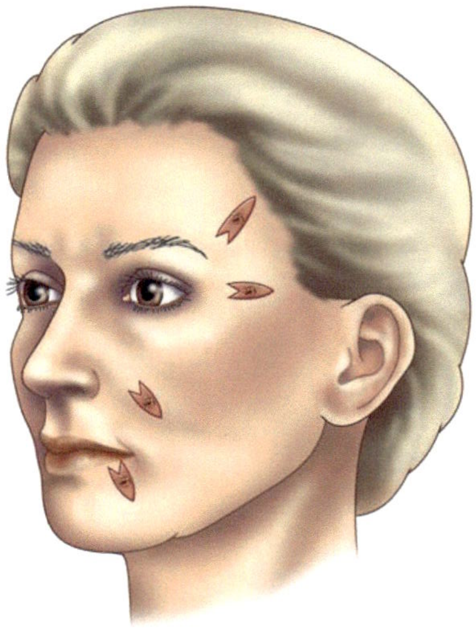

Section C **Advanced Repairs**

Figure 3.5 M-plasty

Section C   **Advanced Repairs**

S-Plasty

When/Where

Mainly used for excision over convex surfaces to decrease contraction and buckling along the length of the scar for better cosmetic result. Common sites for usage include the jaw, shin, and upper extremity.

How

Incise an S-plasty or lazy-S repair by making two S-shaped incisions around the defect. By approximating the center of each slightly offset half the final repair becomes an elongated, serpentine line which contracts over convex surfaces with minimal buckling.

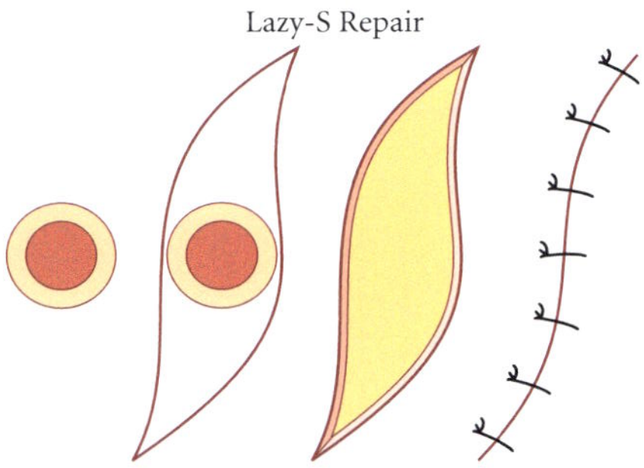

Figure 3.6 S-plasty

Section C Advanced Repairs

Rotation Flap

When/Where
One of the more useful flaps for covering a defect where surrounding skin is loose and flexible. The rotation flap is ideally suited for use on the head and neck.

How
Adjacent tissue is rotated to cover the defect (a slides to meet b); the rotated flap and defect together form a semicircle. The secondary defect created (shaded area, middle, Figure 3.7) may require a free skin graft for closure.

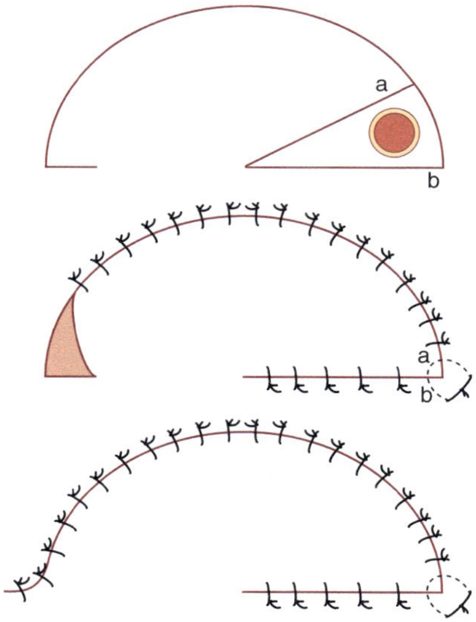

Figure 3.7 Rotation flap

Section C Advanced Repairs

Double Advancement Rotation Flap (O-Z Plasty)

When/Where

Where there is insufficient tissue for a unilateral rotation flap. Because of the Z-formation of the scar, it is preferable not to use this flap on the mid-face area.

How

Advance and rotate flaps to meet each other (a meets b, c meets d). Suture as shown.

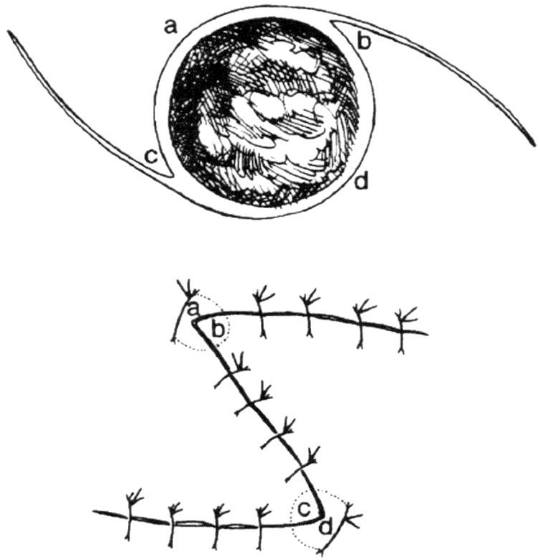

Figure 3.8 Double Rotation Flap

Section C   Advanced Repairs

Rhomboid Flap

When/Where
Basic flap useful in repairing small, circular defects where adjacent tissue is available to rotate onto them.

How
All sides of the triangle and parallelogram should be equal in length (Fig. 3.9A). Undermine and rotate the flap (g slides to meet b, h slides to meet a, f moves into position to be sutured to d). Suture as shown.

Modified Rhomboid: Lengthening all sides of the flap and decreasing the angle at the apex of the secondary defect reduces pivotal restraint and allows for easier closure (Fig. 3.9B).

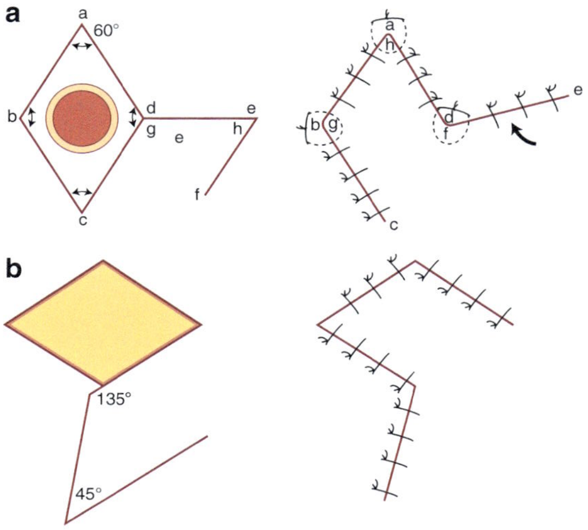

Figure 3.9 Standard rhomboid transposition flap, modified rhomboid flap

Section C   Advanced Repairs

Bilobed Transposition Flap

When/Where

Two transposition flaps in series, useful for repair of defects on the lower 1/3 of the nose between 0.5 and 1.5 cm. Originally described by Esser in 1918, then modified by Zitelli in 1989 by decreasing pivot angle of the flap from 180° to 90–100° which minimizes pincushioning and standing cones at the pivot point.

How

The flap is drawn out with a marker on the skin and then incised, standing cones are removed, and then wide undermining is performed in a submuscular plane. The flap is transposed into position and the tertiary site is closed, next the flap is inset and sutured into the primary defect, and the secondary flap is trimmed and sutured in place.

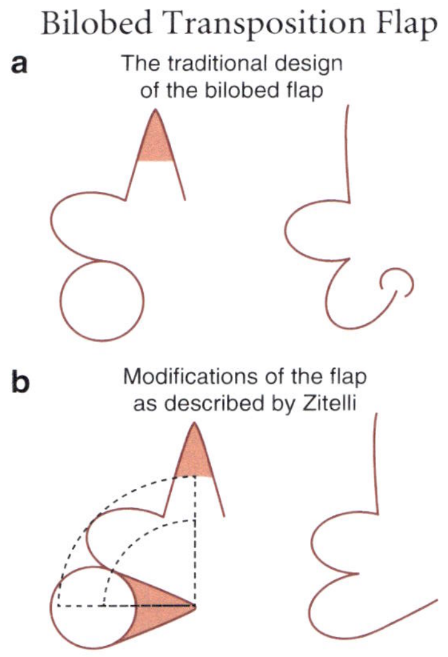

Bilobed Transposition Flap

a The traditional design of the bilobed flap

b Modifications of the flap as described by Zitelli

Figure 3.10 (**a**): Traditional bilobed transposition flap; (**b**): Zitelli modified bilobed transposition flap

Section C   Advanced Repairs

Skin Grafts Overview

Definition—skin and a variable amount of subcutaneous tissue is completely detached from the donor site and sutured into recipient site. For example, full-thickness skin graft, split-thickness skin graft, and composite graft (see Table 3.1)

Stages of Graft Survival

Stage 1: Imbibition—nourishment of graft by plasma, first 24–48 h

Stage 2: Inosculation—graft vessels anastamose, 48 h–10 days

Stage 3: Neovascularization—capillary growth from recipient wound base to graft, circulation reestablished between 4 and 7 days

Stage 4: Maturation—months later, includes reinnervation usually within 2 months, but may take longer or never achieve full sensation

Section C Advanced Repairs

Table 3.1 Skin graft types

	Indications	Donor sites	Advantages	Disadvantages
Full-thickness skin graft: epidermis and full thickness of dermis	Shallow, full thickness facial defects (i.e. medial canthus, helix, nasal tip, and nasal ala)	Preauricular, postauricular, conchal bowl, supraclavicular, nasolabial, and abdomen, inner arm (based on which is best match for recipient site)	Less contraction, retention of appendages, and better color match	Higher metabolic demand, thus more vulnerable to necrosis

(continued)

Section C Advanced Repairs

Table 3.1 (continued)

	Indications	Donor sites	Advantages	Disadvantages
Split-thickness skin graft: epidermis and partial thickness of dermis (0.005–0.03 in.)	Large defects, defects on mucosal surfaces, or for temporary cover of a defect being observed for tumor recurrence	Thighs, buttocks, abdomen, and arms	Best chance of survival, can cover large surface areas, allows wound bed surveillance (for recurrence)	Cosmetically poor, no appendages, poor color match for recipient si
Composite Grafts: epidermis and dermis plus cartilage or other structures	Full thickness defects of nasal ala (loss of cartilage)	Helix of ear, conchal bowl	Restores missing cartilage and maintains better tissue architecture	Highest metabolic demand and failure rate

Section D: Cosmetic Dermatology: Fillers, Neurotoxins, and Chemical Peels

Table 4.1 Botulinum toxin dilutions

Amount of saline used for dilution (mL)	Units of Botox® per 0.1 cc (U)	Common indications
1	10	
2	5	Facial rhytides
2.5	4	Facial rhytides
4	2.5	Axillary hyperhidrosis (usual dose 100 U)
5	2	Axillary hyperhidrosis

Notes:
- Mechanism of action: inhibits acetylcholine (ACh) release by cleaving proteins in the SNARE complex required for ACh release
- Dilution should be performed with 0.9 % normal saline
- One unit of Botox® is approximately equivalent to 2.5–3 units of Dysport® (abobotulinum toxin A)
- One unit of Botox® is approximately equivalent to 1 unit of Xeomin® (incobotulinum toxin A)

Section D: Cosmetic Dermatology: Fillers, Neurotoxins, and Chemical Peels

Table 4.2 Injectable fillers

Filler	Duration	Derivation	Comments
Alloderm®	Months to years	Acellular human cadaveric dermis	Surgically implanted in sterile filed
Artecoll®[a], Artefil®	Permanent (>5 years)	PMMA[b] beads in bovine collagen, allergy test required	Injected deeper than collagen
LaViv®[a]	Months to years	Cultured autologous fibroblasts	Postauricular punch biopsy harvested; cultured by outside laboratory (>3 months)
CosmoDerm®/CosmoPlast®[a]	3–6 months	Human collagen	Products contain lidocaine, no allergy test required

(continued)

Section D Cosmetic Dermatology: Fillers, Neurotoxins, and Chemical Peels

Table 4.2 (continued)

Filler	Duration	Derivation	Comments
Cymetra®[a]	3–6 months	Micronized form of alloderm	Constituted in MD's office, risk for arterial occlusion
DermaLive®/DermaDeep®[a]	Months to years	HA[c] and acrylic hydrogel	Collagen is deposited around minute acrylic particles
Dermalogen®[a]	3–6 months	Pooled human cadaveric collagen	Rarely used
Fat	Variable	Autologous fat and connective tissue	
Gore-Tex®[a]	Permanent	e-PTFE[d]	Injected *below* dermis

(continued)

Section D: Cosmetic Dermatology: Fillers, Neurotoxins, and Chemical Peels

Table 4.2 (continued)

Filler	Duration	Derivation	Comments
Juvederm® Ultra, Ultra Plus, Ultra XC, Juvederm Plus XC[e], Juvederm Voluma	6–12 months, longer for Voluma	HA (bacteria derived)	Juvederm – 18 mg/mL, –24, –30
Belotero®	6 months	HA (bacteria derived)	Fine and superficial rhytides
Perlane®, Perlane- L[e]	6–12 months	HA (bacteria derived)	
Restylane®, Restylane fine lines, Restylane-L, Restylane fine lines-L	6–12 months	HA (bacteria derived)	
Radiesse®	>1 year	Calcium hydroxyapatite/aqueous gel	Formerly known as Radiance
Reviderm®	Months to years	Dextran beads in HA base	

(continued)

Section D Cosmetic Dermatology: Fillers, Neurotoxins, and Chemical Peels

Table 4.2 (continued)

Filler	Duration	Derivation	Comments
Sculptra®	>1 year	Poly-L-lactic acid, dilute with water and lidocaine	FDA approved for HIV—lipodystrophy and aesthetic use
Silicone	Permanent	Manmade polymers	Approved for ophthalmic use
ZyDerm®/ZyPlast®[a]	3–4 months	Bovine collagen	Allergy test required

Filler complications: bleeding/hematoma, swelling, granuloma/nodule formation (if nodules form with hyaluronic acid based filler, consider use of hyaluronidase (off-label, contraindicated if allergic to bee stings)), infection, vascular occlusion, intra-arterial injection (most commonly angular artery and supratrochlear artery) leading to skin necrosis, and scarring, and tyndall effect (especially infraorbital)

[a] Not currently available in the USA
[b] PMMA = polymethylmethacrylate
[c] HA = hyaluronic acid
[d] e-PTFE = expanded polytetrafluoroethylene
[e] These products contain lidocaine; XC=extra comfort, L = lidocaine

Section D: Cosmetic Dermatology: Fillers, Neurotoxins, and Chemical Peels

Table 4.3 Chemical peels

Depth	Commonly used agents	Indications
Superficial	Alpha-hydroxy acids[a] (e.g., citric, glycolic, lactic, malic, mandelic acid, and tartaric acids); Beta-hydroxy acids[b] (e.g., salicylic acid); Jessner's Solution (contains resorcinol, ethanol, lactic acid, and salicylic acid); Trichloroacetic acid <30 %	Epidermal pigmentary disorders, acne and rosacea, and mild photoaging
Medium-depth	Trichloroacetic acid 35–50 % (and combination peels)	Moderate photoaging, actinic keratoses, dyspigmentation, and moderately depressed acne scars
Deep	TCA >50 %, Baker Gordon phenol (need for cardiac monitoring)	Deep rhytides, severe photodamage

Note: consider antiviral prophylaxis if history of orolabial HSV
[a] Alpha-hydroxy acid peels are hydrophilic and must be neutralized
[b] Beta-hydroxy acid peels are lipophilic and thus self-neutralizing

Section E Lasers and Other Technology

Laser Overview: Light Amplification by Stimulated Emission of Radiation

Basic principles

- Laser treatment works by selective photothermolysis: targeted lesion may be destroyed by chromophore absorption of laser light without significant thermal damage to surrounding normal tissue

- Depth of penetration directly proportional to laser wavelength

- Endogenous chromophores: hemoglobin, melanin, and water

- Exogenous chromophores: tattoos

Key terms/units

- J = Joules = Measures of energy

- W = Watts = Measure of power (W = J/s) Fluence (energy density) = J/cm^2

- Irradiance = Power density = W/cm^2

- Thermal relaxation time = Time for structure to cool to 1/2 temperature to which it was heated

E. Hale et al., *Handbook of Dermatologic Surgery*,
10.1007/978-1-4614-8335-9_5, © Springer Science+Business Media New York 2014

Section E Lasers and Other Technology

Table 5.1 Lasers used in dermatology

Laser	Wavelength (nm)/color	Purposes
Carbon dioxide	10,600 (infrared)	Resurfacing, destruction, coagulation, and cutting
Erbium:YAG	2,940 (infrared)	Superficial resurfacing, superficial destruction
Neodynium:YAG	1,064; 1,320 (infrared)	Deep dermal pigmentation, tattoo (black, blue), laser hair removal (LHR), non-ablative resurfacing, large leg veins
Diode	810; 1,450 (infrared)	LHR, acne
Long-pulsed (ms) alexandrite	755 (infrared)	LHR, vascular lesions
Q-switched (ns) alexandrite	755 (infrared)	Tattoo (black, blue, and green), pigmentation

(continued)

Section E Lasers and Other Technology

Table 5.1 (continued)

Laser	Wavelength (nm)/color	Purposes
Picosecond (ps) alexandrite	755 (infrared)	Tattoo (black, blue, and green), pigmented lesions, scars
Q-switched ruby	694 (red)	Pigmentation (epidermal and dermal), tattoo (black, blue, and green), LHR, Nevus of Ota
Argon-pumped tunable red dye	504–690 (green-yellow-red)	Vascular lesions, epidermal pigment

(continued)

Section E Lasers and Other Technology

Table 5.1 (continued)

Laser	Wavelength (nm)/color	Purposes
Flashlamp-pumped dye laser (PDL), long-pulsed pulsed PDL (LP-PDL)	595 (yellow)	Vascular lesions, hypertrophic scars
Flashlamp-pumped yellow dye	585 (yellow)	Vascular lesions, hypertrophic scars, warts
Copper vapor/bromide	578 (yellow), 511 (green)	Vascular lesions, epidermal pigment
Krypton	568 (yellow), 521/531 (green)	Vascular lesions, epidermal pigment

(continued)

Section E   Lasers and Other Technology

Table 5.1 (continued)

Laser	Wavelength (nm)/color	Purposes
KTP (potassium titanyl phosphate)	532 (green)	Vascular lesions, epidermal pigment
Q-switched (frequency doubled) Nd:YAG	532 (green)	Vascular lesions, epidermal pigment, red tattoo
Argon continuous (gas)	514 (green), 488 (blue)	Vascular lesions, epidermal pigment
Flashlamp-pumped green dye	504, 510 (green)	Epidermal pigment, red tattoo
Pulsed excimer	193, 308, 351 (UV)	Psoriasis, vitiligo, LASIK

Section E   Lasers and Other Technology

Table 5.2 Fractionated laser devices

Type	Wavelength (nm)	Brand name
Ablative devices		
CO_2	10,600	Fraxel Re:pair®, SmartSkin®, SmartXide DOT®, UltraPulse®, Deep FX®
Erbium-YAG	2,940	Lux 2940®, Pixel®, Pro-fractional®
YSGG	2,790	Pearl fractional®
Non-ablative devices		
Erbium/Thulium	1,550, 1,927	Fraxel Dual®

(continued)

Section E Lasers and Other Technology

Table 5.2 (continued)

Type	Wavelength (nm)	Brand name
Erbium fiber	1,550	Fraxel Re:store®
Erbium fiber	1,410	Fraxel Re:fine®
Diode	1,440, 1,927	Clear and Brilliant®
Erbium:Glass	1,540	Fractional 1540®, Mosaic®, Matisse®
Nd-YAG	1,440, 1,320	Affirm®

Note: fluences and pulse widths vary among above

Section E   Lasers and Other Technology

Table 5.3 Home use and low-energy devices

Type	Wavelength (nm)	Indication
Fractional non-ablative	1,410, 1,435	Periorbital rhytids
Diode	655, 650	Androgenetic alopecia
Diode	810	Hair removal (brown and black hairs)
IPL (intense pulsed light)	475–1,200	Hair removal (brown and black hairs)
IPL	400–1,100	Acne
IPL	480–2,000	Acne
nbUVB[a]	300–320	Psoriasis

(continued)

Section E Lasers and Other Technology

Table 5.3 (continued)

Type	Wavelength (nm)	Indication
Heat	NA	Acne, hair removal
Heat	NA	Acne
Heat	NA	Hair removal
LED[b]-blue	414, 415	Acne
LED-red and blue	415, 633	Acne
LED-red	660	Periorbital rhytids

[a] nb=narrowband
[b] LED=light emitting diode

Section E Lasers and Other Technology

Table 5.4 Tattoo removal by laser

Tattoo color	Pigments used	Lasers used
Red	Mercuric sulfide, Cadmium selenide, and Sienna	QS[a] Nd:YAG 532 nm, Pulsed-dye 510 nm
Green	Chromates malachite, Ferro-ferric cyanide phthalocyanine dyes curcuma	QS Ruby 694 nm, QS Alexandrite 755 nm, [b]PS Alexandrite 755 nm
Black and dark-blue	Carbon, Iron oxide, and logwood	QS Ruby 694 nm, QS Alexandrite 755 nm
		Nd:YAG 1,064 nm, PS Alexandrite 755 nm
Light blue	Cobalt	PS Alexandrite 755 nm
Yellow (hard to treat)	Cadmium sulfide	QS Nd-YAG 532 nm

(continued)

Section E Lasers and Other Technology

Table 5.4 (continued)

Tattoo color	Pigments used	Lasers used
Brown	Iron oxide	QS Nd-YAG 532 nm, QS Ruby 694 nm, QS Nd-YAG 1,064 nm, QS Alexandrite 755 nm
White	Titanium	QS Nd-YAG 532 nm

Note: Caution treating tattoos containing white pigment (white, peach, pink, and flesh-toned tattoos), as there is a risk of paradoxical darkening due to reduction of ferric oxide to ferrous oxide

[a]QS = Q-switched: nanosecond pulses of energy (10^{-9} s)
[b]PS = picosecond (10^{-12} s)

Section E Lasers and Other Technology

Table 5.5 Photo-induced eye injury

Wavelength (nm)	Absorbed by	Method of injury
UVB & UVC (100–320)	Cornea (photokeratitis)	Sunburn
UVA (320–400)	Lens (cataract)	PUVA
Visible (400–700)	Retina (melanin, photoreceptors), pigmented retinal epithelium	Ruby, pulsed dye, and argon lasers
Near-infrared and Infrared (700+)	Cornea, retina	CO_2, Er:YAG, Nd:YAG lasers

Note: When operating lasers ensure to wear wrap-around glasses and goggles with adequate optical density for given wavelength of laser. Ensure patients' eyes are shielded adequately

Section E Lasers and Other Technology

Novel Devices: Skin Tightening and Body Sculpting

Radiofrequency Devices: monopolar radiofrequency (RF) energy generates heat which produces collagen contraction after disruption of hydrogen bonds of collagen helix. For example, ThermaCool TC® (Thermage). FDA approved for periorbital rhytid reduction, also commonly used for skin tightening on face/neck. Bipolar RF devices create localized heat by conducting current between the two electrodes on the skin surface.

Focused Ultrasound Devices: based on theoretical principal that intense ultrasound field vibrates tissue creating friction between molecules causing them to absorb mechanical energy and leading to secondary generation of heat. Heating of the fat tissue due to the absorption of acoustic energy leads to immediate tissue contraction and delayed collagen remodeling with the coagulative change limited to the focal region of the ultrasound field. Technology is used for noninvasive body sculpting/contouring. For example, Ulthera® (FDA approved), LipoSonix® (FDA approved).

Cryolipolysis: Targeted production of adipocyte apoptosis via thermal energy extraction by cooling (without damage to the epidermis). For example, CoolSculpting (Zeltiq®) (FDA approved).

Section F Leg Veins

Leg Vein Treatment Overview

- Superficial telangiectasia (pink, red, <1 mm), reticular veins (blue, green, 1–3 mm), and varicose veins (blue, green, colorless, >3 mm) of the lower extremities are interconnected and commonly develop after impairment of venous return due to valvular incompetence.

- Prior to treatment, a comprehensive history should be taken with particular attention to family history of varicose veins, prior venous procedures, coagulopathy, anticipated immobility or travel, pregnancy/lactation, concurrent minocycline therapy (due to risk of long-lasting pigmentary alteration), arterial insufficiency, migraine with aura, patent foramen ovale (PFO), and presence of venous symptoms (see below).

- Consider duplex ultrasound if bulging varicose veins within zones of influence of saphenous systems or presence of signs/symptoms of superficial venous insufficiency, including swelling, aching, burning, restless legs, cramping, stasis dermatitis, ulceration, or lipodermatosclerosis.

- Sclerotherapy remains the gold standard for treatment of non-varicose leg veins.

Section F Leg Veins

- Detergent solutions (see Table 6.2) can be combined with air (1:3–4) and agitated via a two- or three-way stop-cock in order to create foam—Tessari method.

- Foam sclerotherapy (which is not FDA approved) can be used for treatment of large networks of vessels, and is particularly useful for duplex guided sclerotherapy due to its echogenicity. There is an increased risk of adverse side effects, including visual disturbances and transient CNS events. Use should be avoided in patients with a known patent foramen ovale (PFO).

- Proximal reflux/larger veins should be treated before related small veins.

- Treatments should be spaced approximately 6 weeks apart.

- Most common side effects are ecchymosis, postsclerotherapy pigmentation (more common with higher concentrations and after foam sclerotherapy), matting, and ulceration.

- Postoperative compression improves efficacy of vein treatments, reduces risk of thromboembolism, reduces risk of pigmentation (due to intravascular coagulum formation), and increases the rate of recovery, although optimal duration of compression is unclear.

- Laser treatment is an option for patients with severe needle phobia or recalcitrant vessels (see Table 6.1).

Section F Leg Veins

Leg Vein Treatment Algorithm

1. Saphenous incompetence (see Figs. 1.15 and 1.16)

    (a) Ablation (endovenous laser/radiofrequency), ligation +/− short stripping

    (b) Duplex-guided foam sclerotherapy

2. Saphenous branches

    (a) Ambulatory phlebectomy

    (b) Duplex-guided foam sclerotherapy

3. Reticular veins

    (a) Sclerotherapy (foam or liquid)

    (b) Laser (see Table 6.1)

    (c) Ambulatory phlebectomy

4. Venulectasia and telangiectatic spider veins

    (a) Sclerotherapy

    (b) Laser (see Table 6.1)

Section F: Leg Veins

Table 6.1 Laser for leg veins

Type of vessel	Laser/wavelength
Small, superficial, and red vessels (<1 mm in diameter and depth)	KTP 532 nm, PDL 585–595 nm, and IPL (500–1,200)
Large, deep vessels (>1 mm in diameter and depth)	Alexandrite 755 nm, Diode 800–980 nm, and Nd:YAG 1,064 nm
Axial or truncal varicosities	Endovenous lasers: Diode (810, 940, and 980 nm), Infrared (1,319, 1,320, and 1,470 nm), and radiofrequency

Note:
- Larger blood vessels need longer pulse durations (10–50 ms)
- Spot size diameter should be approximately 1–2× the size of the vessel
- Type III skin and above should only be treated with infrared wavelengths
- Avoid pulse stacking and aggressively cool when utilizing infrared lasers

Section F Leg Veins

Table 6.2 Sclerotherapy agents

Agent	Brand names	Type	FDA approved	Comments
Hypertonic saline (HS, 11.7–23.4 %)	None	Hyperosmolar	Yes (use for sclerotherapy is off-label)	Low risk of allergy; highly ulcerogenic with extravasation; and painful cramping and burning
HS + Dextrose	Sclerodex	Hyperosmolar	No	Low risk of allergy
72 % glycerin[a]	None	Hyperosmolar	Yes (use for sclerotherapy is off-label)	Low risk of pigmentation; weak sclerosant; must be specially compounded

(continued)

Section F Leg Veins

Table 6.2 (continued)

Agent	Brand names	Type	FDA approved	Comments
Sodium tetradecyl sulfate (STS)	Sotradecol, FibroVein, Trombovar, and Thromboject	Detergent	Yes	Painless intravascular injection; ulcerogenic if extravasation (>0.25 %), expensive
Polidocanol	Asclera, Aethoxysklerol, Sclero-Vein	Detergent	Yes	Painless (polidocanol is an anesthetic); low risk of extravasation necrosis; causes injection site urticaria; expensive
Sodium morrhuate	Scleromate	Detergent	Yes[b]	Highest anaphylaxis risk; no longer used

(continued)

Section F Leg Veins

Table 6.2 (continued)

Agent	Brand names	Type	FDA approved	Comments
Ethanolamine oleate	Ethamolin	Detergent	Yes[b]	Primarily used for esophageal varices; not used for leg veins
Chromated glycerin	Sclermo, Chromex	Chemical irritant	No[b]	Used widely in Europe
Sodium salicylate		Chemical irritant	No[b]	Rarely if ever used
Polyiodinated iodine	Variglobin, clerodine, and iodo-Ioduree	Chemical irritant	No[b]	High necrosis risk; rarely if ever used

[a]Typically compounded 2:1 with 1 % plain lidocaine or 1 % lidocaine with epinephrine
[b]Rarely, if ever used in USA

Index

A
Adson forceps, 68
Aspirin, 18

B
Bilateral advancement flap, 91
Bilobed transposition flap, 89
Bishop Harmon forceps, 69
Buried vertical mattress stitch, 44

C
Castroviejo needle driver, 73
Chalazion clamp, 74
Chondritis, 61
Composite graft, 92
Contact dermatitis, 60
Cosmetic dermatology
 Botox dilutions, 93
 chemical peels, 98
 injectable fillers, 94–97
Cranial nerve V branches, 4, 5
Cryolipolysis, 111
Cryosurgery, 30–31
Curved Mayo scissor, 72
Cutaneous flap
 advancement flap
  bilateral advancement flap, 91
  M-plasty, 83–84
  single advancement flap, 80
  S-plasty, 85
  Z-plasty, 82
 axial flap, 79
 bilobed transposition flap, 89
 random pattern, 79
 rhomboid flap, 88
 rotation flap, 86–87
 staged flap, 79
Cutaneous vertical mattress stitch, 45

Index

D
Dabigatran etexilate, 19
Dog ear repair
  excision line elongation, 50
  leashing, 51–52
  wound closure, 50
Double advancement rotation flap (O-Z plasty), 87

E
Electrosurgery, 28–29, 60
Epinephrine, 26
Esters, 24–25
Excessive granulation tissue, 62
Excisional and non-excisional surgery
  anesthetics
    local, 23–26
    topical, 26
    tumescent solution, 27
  anticoagulants
    antiseptic scrubs, 22
    aspirin, 18
    dabigatran etexilate, 19
    thienopyridine, 18
    warfarin, 18–19
  Castroviejo needle driver, 73
  Chalazion clamp, 74
  cryosurgery, 30–31
  curettes, 66
  dog ear repair
    excision line elongation, 50
    leashing, 51–52
    wound closure, 50
  electrosurgery, 28–29
  elliptical fusiform excision, 41
  english nail splitter, 76
  facial incisions and excisions, 42
  forceps
    Adson forceps, 68
    Bishop Harmon forceps, 69
    Jacobson hemostat forceps, 70
  medical history, 17
  melanoma staging, 34–37
  Mohs micrographic surgery
    indications, 38
    procedure, 39–40

Index

nail elevator, 77
needle holders, 67
prophylactic and empiric antibiotics, 20–21
scalpel blades, 65
scalpel handles, 64
scissors, 71–72
skin hooks, 75
stitches
   buried vertical mattress stitch, 44
   cutaneous vertical mattress stitch, 45
   horizontal mattress stitch, 46
   pulley stitch, 48
   running subcuticular stitch, 47
   simple interrupted stitch, 43
surgical margins, 32–33
suture
   absorbable sutures, 53–54
   nonabsorbable sutures, 55
   removal timetable, 34–37
   spitting, 61
   three point suture, 49
   track marks, 61

topical antimicrobial agents, 56–57
wound dressing, 58
External ear, anatomy, 9
Eye, anatomy, 10

F

Face
   nerve branches, 4, 5
   skin tension lines, 12
   subunits of, 8
   vascular supply, 5
Foam sclerotherapy, 114
Full-thickness skin graft, 91

H

Head and neck muscle anatomy, 3
Horizontal mattress stitch, 46
H-plasty, 91
Hydrocolloids, 58
Hydrogel, 58
Hyperpigmented scars, 62

Index

Hypertrophic scars and keloids, 62
Hypopigmented scars, 62

I
Infections, 60
Interface protector, 58

J
Jacobson hemostat forceps, 70

L
Laser treatment
  fractionated laser devices, 104–105
  home use and low-energy devices, 106–107
  photo-induce eye injury, 110
  principles, 99
  skin tightening and body sculpting, 111
  tattoo removal, 108–109
  types, 100–103
Leg vein treatment
  algorithm, 115
  comprehensive history, 113
  duplex ultrasound, 113
  laser, 114, 116
  sclerotherapy
    agents, 114, 117–119
    postoperative compression, 114
    side effects, 114
    superficial telangiectasia, 113
Lidocaine, 25–26

M
Metzenbaum scissor with blunted tips, 72
Mohs micrographic surgery
  indications, 38
  procedure, 39–40
M-plasty, 83–84

N
Nail unit, anatomy, 11
Nose, anatomy, 7

Index

O
O-Z plasty, 87

P
Photo-induce eye injury, 110
Polyurethane films and foams, 58
Prophylactic antibiotics, 21
Pulley stitch, 48

R
Rhomboid flap, 88
Rotation flap, 86–87
Running subcuticular/intradermal stitch, 47

S
Saphenous vein, 15–16
Sensory nerves, face, 4
Single advancement flap, 80
Single tangent advancement flap, 80

Skin grafts
 definition, 90
 survival stages, 90
 types, 91–92
Skin necrosis, 61
Skin tension lines
 anterior, 13
 face, 12
 posterior, 14
Skull
 anterior view, 1
 lateral view, 2
S-plasty, 85
Split-thickness skin graft, 92
Surgical anatomy
 external ear, 9
 eye, 10
 face
  nerve branches, 4, 5
  sensory nerves, 4
  skin tension lines, 12
  subunits of, 8

Index

Surgical anatomy (*cont.*)
    vascular supply, 5
head and neck muscle, 3
nails, 11
nose, 7
saphenous vein, 15–16
skin tension lines, 12–14
skull
    anterior view, 1
    lateral view, 2
Suture spitting, 61

T
Thienopyridine, 18

V
Vertical mattress stitch
    buried, 44
    cutaneous, 45

W
Warfarin, 18–19

Z
Z-plasty, 82